Substance Abuse
During Pregnancy and Childhood

Drug and Alcohol Abuse Reviews

Edited by

Ronald R. Watson

Drug and Alcohol Abuse Reviews • 8

Substance Abuse During Pregnancy and Childhood

Edited by

Ronald R. Watson

University of Arizona, Tucson, Arizona

Humana Press • Totowa, New Jersey

This publication is printed on acid-free paper. ∞
ANSI Z39.48-1984 (American National Standards Institute)
Permanence of Paper for Printed Library Materials.

Photocopy Authorization Policy:
Authorization to photocopy items for internal or personal use, or the internal or personal use of specific clients, is granted by Humana Press Inc., provided that the base fee of US $4.00 per copy, plus US $00.20 per page, is paid directly to the Copyright Clearance Center at 222 Rosewood Drive, Danvers, MA 01923. For those organizations that have been granted a photocopy license from the CCC, a separate system of payment has been arranged and is acceptable to Humana Press Inc. The fee code for users of the Transactional Reporting Service is: [0-89603-295-7/95 $4.00 + $00.20].

Printed in the United States of America. 9 8 7 6 5 4 3 2 1
Library of Congress Cataloging-in-Publication Data

Substance abuse during pregnancy and childhood/edited by Ronald R. Watson.
    p. cm.—(Drug and alcohol abuse reviews; 8)
  Includes index.
  ISBN 0-89603-295-7 (alk. paper)
  1. Substance abuse in pregnancy—Prevention. 2. Fetal alcohol syndrome—Prevention. 3. Teenage girls—Alcohol use. 4. Teenage girls—Drug use.
I. Watson, Ronald R. (Ronald Ross)   II. Series.
  [DNLM: 1. Substance Abuse—in pregnancy. 2. Alcoholism. 3. Maternal–Fetal Exchange. 4. Substance Abuse—prevention & control. WM 270
  D79358   1995]
RG580.S75D784 1995
618.3'268—dc20
DNLM/DLC   94-44482
for Library of Congress   CIP

Contents

Preface

Alcohol and other drugs of abuse cause significant physiological changes, especially during development. The effects on the infant and child range from severe mental retardation to mild changes in activity and neurological functions. Although the level of intake needed to cause fetal damage is not clear, the magnitude of the problem is significant, with many long-term sequelae.

As a result, it becomes critical to better diagnose and manage drug and alcohol use during pregnancy. This must involve special training for health care professionals. In addition, recognition of the psychosocial factors affecting alcohol use, especially by youth and young adults, is critical to modifying behavior, and thus reducing fetal alcohol exposure.

Cultural considerations can also come into play in modifying alcohol and drug use by women so as to reduce fetal damage. The trends in alcohol and drug use by youth forecast rising levels of damage to infants. These children will need extensive medical and educational care for years to decades.

Clearly, understanding of the role women must take in modifying their alcohol and drug use during pregnancy will facilitate changes in our cultural and educational practices that will help reduce fetal trauma from alcohol.

Ronald R. Watson

Contributors

Luis B. Curet • *Department of Obstetrics and Gynecology, University of New Mexico, Albuquerque, NM*

Kathleen J. Farkas • *Mandel School of Applied Social Sciences, Case Western Reserve University, Cleveland, OH*

Meg Gerrard • *Department of Psychology, Iowa State University, Ames, IA*

Frederick X. Gibbons • *Department of Psychology, Iowa State University, Ames, IA*

Tami J. Hedges • *Department of Psychology, Iowa State University, Ames, IA*

R. J. Russac • *Department of Psychology, University of North Florida, Jacksonville, FL*

Gabie E. Smith • *Department of Psychology, Iowa State University, Ames, IA*

Vivian L. Smith • *Center for Substance Abuse Prevention, US Department of Health and Human Services, Rockville, MD*

Sharon T. Weaver • *College of Health, University of North Florida, Jacksonville, FL*

Diagnosis and Management of Drug Abuse During Pregnancy

Assessment of Consequences

Luis B. Curet

Introduction

Substance abuse during pregnancy is an enormous problem with staggering medical and social relevance. Although there are extensive data on illicit drug use by nonpregnant women, it is problematic to translate that data in order to estimate drug use by pregnant women. Using selected studies[1] the National Association for Perinatal Addiction Research and Education has estimated that 375,000 infants are born each year to mothers who abuse drugs.[2] The figure is higher if alcohol is included. Based on this estimate and reports from various programs, it appears that the incidence of illicit drug

From: *Drug and Alcohol Abuse Reviews, Vol. 8:*
Drug and Alcohol Abuse During Pregnancy and Childhood
Ed.: R. R. Watson ©1995 Humana Press Inc., Totowa, NJ

use during pregnancy is around 10%. At the University of New Mexico Medical Center, 7% of pregnant women tested positive for illicit drugs in the urine on presentation to the labor and delivery unit.

Late or no prenatal care is common among pregnant drug users.[3] Vaginal bleeding and preterm labor are also associated with increased drug use. Other markers for increased risk of substance abuse are a history of physical and sexual abuse, drug use by parents, and tobacco use. It is of interest that the rate of substance abuse during pregnancy among Black women is not different than Whites.

The problems of drug exposure by pregnant women and their children are multifactorial, with a particular drug presenting only one factor. Polydrug use now appears to be the norm. Problems also occur with maternal nutrition; access to medical care, including prenatal care; finances; family stability; and psychological issues, such as low self-esteem. The typical personality profile is one of low self-confidence; poor coping skills; multiple social, family, and personal problems; depression; and anxiety. They may suffer from psychiatric problems, such as mood disorders, schizophrenia, passive-aggressive, and antisocial behaviors.[4]

Thus, the care of substance-abusing pregnant women is not simple. A treatment plan that deals with all these problems must be implemented in order to modify the pregnant woman's behavior, keep her free of drugs, and help her deal with the issues contributing or predisposing her to continue using drugs.

Comprehensive Programs

It has been shown that comprehensive treatment programs for pregnant substance abusers are successful.[5] Such programs must include obstetric and pediatric care, parenting classes, home visits, and substance abuse treatment. Additionally, vocational rehabilitation, childcare, childbirth preparation, and education must be addressed. Such services must address the specific needs of the women and must reduce barriers to recovery.

Referral into such a comprehensive program depends to a great degree on the ability of the physician to identify the addiction characteristics of pregnant women. The diagnosis of substance abuse during pregnancy is frequently missed. Chasnoff[6] stated that the reported incidence of substance abuse in pregnancy depends on the thoroughness of the assessment by the health care provider. If the referring physician is able to identify the pregnant patient with a substance abuse problem, he or she can be instrumental in promoting the overall health of both the woman and the infant.

Identification

Knowledge of the medical, historical, and behavioral characteristics that help identify addicted pregnant women is of paramount importance. In addition, there are a number of instruments that have had their reliability established and should be used during the intake process.

The following historical indicators suggest substance dependence:[7]

1. Drug-abusing partner;
2. Narcotic withdrawal symptom in a previous neonate;
3. Previous infants with low birth weight and poor perinatal outcomes;
4. Family history of substance abuse;
5. History of sudden infant death syndrome;
6. Disrupted family; and
7. Affective disorders.

The following behavioral indicators should also alert the provider:

1. Domestic violence;
2. History of child and/or sexual abuse;
3. Depression;
4. Unreliable, inappropriate, or unpredictable behavior;
5. Chronic unemployment; and
6. Intoxicated behavior.

Medical indicators include:

1. Poor nutritional status;
2. HIV positive test;
3. Hepatitis;
4. Multiple abscesses;
5. Withdrawal symptoms;
6. Irregular menstruation;
7. Tuberculosis;
8. Sexually transmitted diseases; and
9. Obstetrical complications like abruptio placenta, preterm labor, absent or erratic prenatal care, and premature rupture of membranes.

Urine testing is part of the identification process. However, it can be misleading because most drugs have a short half-life and frequently urine samples will be negative, even though it is obvious, by her behavior, the patient has been using drugs.

It is also unsuccessful to try to elicit specific substance abuse behavior during the early phases of treatment. It is first necessary to build an alliance with the patient, and, after rapport is firmly established, to then question the patient about specific behavior. In our program, we have delayed specific interviewing until the second or third visit, or later if necessary, to allow the patient to voluntarily provide us with an account of her behavior. It is important to remember that most patients are unwilling to divulge information about drug-using behavior, even though most people do admit to smoking and drinking, although seldom to excessive use of such socially acceptable drugs. Even women who admit to substance use during pregnancy underestimate their use.

Because even limited use of alcohol and other drugs has teratogenic potential, questionnaire instruments can be helpful as they measure not only addiction but also sporadic use. Instruments that have been proven to be reliable include the Drug and Alcohol History,[7] the Ten Question Drinking history,[8] and the Michigan Alcoholism Screening Test (MAST),[9] all of which are widely used. Other instruments that may be useful include the Drug Abuse Screening Test (DAST),[10] the CAGE Questionnaire,[11] and the History of Trauma Scale.[12] These instruments were designed to assess the presence and extent of substance use and abuse. It has not been clearly demonstrated, however, that the cutoff points for these tests apply equally well to pregnant women of diverse ethnic and cultural backgrounds.

Based on studies that demonstrate the effectiveness of early detection and intervention,[1] screening guidelines should:

1. Promote the goal of prenatal identification as improving care rather than punishing. Thus, a nonjudgmental approach is of the utmost importance.
2. Emphasize that pregnant women should be routinely asked about tobacco and alcohol use and, at the appropriate time, about illegal drug use.
3. Include use of appropriate instruments to complement history intake.
4. Promote alertness for behavioral, physical, and psychosocial signs and symptoms of substance-seeking behavior.
5. Include the use of urine testing, even though it remains debatable and needs individualization to specific patients.

Treatment

The comprehensive care required by pregnant substance abusers is not yet widely accepted. At the University of New

Mexico-School of Medicine, we have implemented such a program under the name of MILAGRO. This is the Spanish translation of the word "miracle." The MILAGRO program is centered around the prenatal clinic which is housed in a separate building from the general OB clinic. The clinic serves as the center of activities for the pregnant women in the program.

The following services are provided at the clinic:

1. Couples and family therapy;
2. Home visits;
3. Childbirth classes;
4. Individual counseling;
5. Infant massage classes;
6. Group therapy;
7. Prenatal care;
8. Hospital visits;
9. Psychiatric supervision;
10. Methadone meetings;
11. Childcare;
12. Parenting classes; and
13. Methadone dispensing.

A residential program in close proximity to the clinic allows for more intensive care of selected patients. Additional services provided specifically for patients in the residential hall include:

1. Narcotics Anonymous (NA) meetings;
2. Childcare;
3. Play time;
4. Menu planning, meal preparation, and nutritional classes;
5. Free time for self-determined activities;
6. Women's support group;
7. Exercise;
8. Grocery shopping;
9. Psycho-educational group therapy;

10. Yoga class;
11. Meetings with welfare, probation, and other agencies;
12. Patient outings; and
13. Family visitation.

Linkages with a number of agencies and providers have been established so that patients can access a number of services, including acupuncture, AA, vocational rehabilitation, mental health services, and others.

All infants born to patients are followed in a special pediatric clinic staffed by both MILAGRO and Department of Health personnel. In addition to routine pediatric care, neurologic and psychomotor evaluations are performed every 1–6 mo. After delivery, patients remain in the MILAGRO Program until 6–12 mo, when their care is gradually transferred to the women's program of the Center for Alcoholism Substance Abuse and Addiction (CASAA), which is one of the organizations working closely with MILAGRO.

Specific emphasis is placed on the consequences of maternal drug use on both mother and baby. Although these are well known to providers, many of the patients are not fully aware of such effects and intensive education is required. Congenital anomalies and deficiencies in fetal growth are relatively easy to diagnose at birth. It is developmental delays, abnormalities in cognitive functioning, and behavioral abnormalities associated with *in utero* exposure to drugs that require careful assessment. Thus, treatment programs must use carefully tested instruments to evaluate both the effects of drug use and treatment.

The Stanford Binet Intelligence Scale, designed to measure intelligence, regarded as general mental adaptability, has been used by many investigators and found to be reliable. However, one must be careful and consider the ethnic and cultural characteristics of the population studied when using the age standards of performance. The McCarthy Scales, likewise, evaluate cognitive ability. Its general cognitive index correlates well with the Stanford Binet IQ.

The Kaufman Assessment Battery for Children was designed to evaluate children's intelligence and achievement. Factors that affect the total score include language concepts, school-related skills, and knowledge of facts. Unfortunately, these factors are affected by many other parameters besides drug use and treatment. Still, many investigators prefer this instrument to the Wide Range Achievement Test and the California Achievement Test because it gives a measure of the child's exposure to and retention of environmental detail, and an indication of the child's ability to arrive at a conclusion when given several facts. Additionally, it provides a measure of reading comprehension.[3]

The Roberts Apperception Test for children allows for an assessment of children's perceptions, which aids in evaluating the child's personality. It uses a simple and objective scoring system. The various scales permit the identification of specific problem areas.[13]

The Bayley Scales of Infant Development have been extensively used by many investigators. The various scales have been shown to provide reliable evaluation scores[14] for assessment of psychomotor, mental, and behavioral development. At the MILAGRO Program we have used the Bayley and have found it to be compatible with the cultural and ethnic background of our patients. It has seemed better for us to use one instrument and become very familiar with it as opposed to using a multiplicity of assessment instruments.

The Neonatal Behavioral Assessment Scale is the most frequently used instrument to assess neurobehavior of the neonate. This behavior, although reflecting genetic makeup, also reflects intrauterine exposures. Neonates exposed *in utero* to drugs are more irritable, less cuddly, more tremulous, and show more hypertonicity than nonexposed neonates.[15] The neonates also appear to be less responsive to usual stimulation.

Our data and that of other investigators[13,14] show significant differences between infants of drug-using women and controls. The study by Hans[14] is of interest in that methadone-exposed infants lagged behind comparison infants in physical growth and motor functioning as well as cognitive development.

The effects of prenatal use of heroin/methadone are usually quantitated by the severity of neonatal withdrawal. We use an abstinence scoring system based on presence and severity of gastrointestinal, metabolic, vasomotor, and central nervous system signs. Elevated scores are indications for treatment. Although treatment with paregoric, phenobarbital, or tincture of opium is frequently used, we have found that treatment with methadone is quite effective.

After delivery we observe the neonate for a minimum of 96 h. During the observation period, the withdrawal scoring system is utilized. The scoring starts 24 h postnatally and continues as long as the neonate shows signs of withdrawal. In general, when the neonate has a score of 5–8, efforts are made to assist with self-regulation. If the score is ≥8 pharmacologic management with low-dose methadone is started. Scoring for signs of withdrawal continues until the baby has weaned off entirely. This process can take from 7 d to 6 wk.

A 2-kg infant receiving 0.7 mg/kg/24 h would be weaned as follows:

Day 1   0.250 mg every 4 h
Day 2   0.125 mg every 4 h
Day 3   0.125 mg every 6 h
Day 4   0.125 mg every 8 h
Day 5   0.125 mg every 12 h
Day 6   0.0625 mg every 12 h
Day 7   0.0625 mg daily or twice a day

Dose intervals are only a guide and the schedule may be individualized.

De Cubas and Field,[13] in a study of 20 children exposed to methadone *in utero* and 20 controls, found no differences in cognitive functioning. However, the IQ scores of children showing evidence of withdrawal at birth were lower than those of asymptomatic children. In spite of the lower IQ scores, the methadone children functioned at grade level. Other investigators[14–18] have reported no differences during infancy. However, fewer studies have followed these children past infancy. In view of the fact that the infant's environment has a significant effect on development and that the lifestyle of drug-using women differs from nondrug users, it would be extremely difficult to identify prenatal exposure as the sole cause of developmental impairment.

As Lawson and Wilson[19] stated, narcotic dependent women are poorly equipped for their maternal role. They attempt to provide parenting to infants who are extremely difficult to care for. Therefore, the significance of prenatal exposure to drugs should be seen as a stage in a continuum of risk factors, and its relative importance is still in need of complete elucidation.

References

[1]S. F. Wheeler (1993) Substance abuse during pregnancy. *Primary Care* **20**, 191–207.

[2]S. Silverman (1989) Scope, specifics of maternal drug use, effects on fetus are beginning to emerge from studies. *JAMA* **261**, 1688,1689.

[3]L. P. Finnegan (1991) Perinatal substance abuse: comments and perspectives. *Semin. Perinatal.* **15**, 331–339.

[4]I. J. Chasnoff (1988) *Drugs, Alcohol, Pregnancy and Parenting.* Kluwer Academic, Hingham, MA.

[5]F. Suffet and R. Brotman (1984) A comprehensive care program for pregnant addicts: obstetrical, neonatal, and child development outcomes. *Int. J. Addict.* **19**, 199–219.

[6]I. J. Chasnoff (1989) Drug use and women: establishing a standard of care. *Ann. NY Acad. Sci.* **562,** 208–210.

[7]M. Jessup (1990) The treatment of perinatal addiction: identification, intervention and advocacy. *West J. Med.* **152,** 553–558.

[8]H. L. Rosett, L. Weiner, and K. C. Edelin (1983) Treatment experience with pregnant problem drinkers. *JAMA* **249,** 2029–2033.

[9]M. L. Selzer (1971) Michigan Alcoholism Screening Test. *Am. J. Psychiatry* **127,** 1653–1658.

[10]H. Skinner (1982) The Drug Abuse Screening Test. *Addict. Behav.* **7,** 363–371.

[11]J. A. Ewing (1984) Detecting alcoholism: the CAGE Questionnaire. *JAMA* **252,** 1905–1907.

[12]H. A. Skinner, S. Holt, R. Schuller, J. Roy, and Y. Israel (1984) Identification of alcohol abuse using laboratory tests and a history of trauma. *Ann. Int. Med.* **101,** 847–851.

[13]M. M. De Cubas and T. Field (1993) Children of methadone-dependent women: developmental outcomes. *Am. J. Orthopsych.* **63,** 266–276.

[14]S. L. Hans (1989) Developmental consequences of prenatal exposure to methadone. *Ann. NY Acad. Sci.* **562,** 195–207.

[15]K. A. Kaltenbach and L. Finnegan (1989) Prenatal narcotic exposure: perinatal and developmental effects. *Neurotoxicology* **10,** 597–604.

[16]A. Lodge (1977) *Developmental Findings with Infants Born to Mothers on Methadone Maintenance.* A preliminary report edited by G. Beschner and R. B. Rothman. Symposium on Comprehensive Health Care for Addicted Families and Their children, Government Printing Office, Washington, DC.

[17]M. E. Strauss, J. S. Lessen-Firestone, C. J. Chavez, and J. C. Stryker (1979) Children of methadone treated women at five years of age. *Pharmacol. Bioch. Behav. Suppl.* **11,** 3–6.

[18]G. S. Wilson, M. M. Desmond, and R. B. Wait (1981) Follow up of methadone treated women and their infants: health, developmental and social implications. *J. Pediatr.* **98,** 716–722.

[19]M. S. Lawson and G. S. Wilson (1980) Parenting among women addicted to narcotics. *Child Med.* **2,** 67–79.

Training Health Care and Human Services Personnel in Perinatal Substance Abuse

Kathleen J. Farkas

Introduction

Perinatal substance abuse treatment is composed of overlapping areas: maternal and child health care, alcohol and other drug abuse treatment, child abuse prevention, and domestic violence prevention. The field of perinatal substance abuse lies at the intersection of the complex social, medical, and psychological needs of women who abuse substances before, during, and/or after pregnancy, and the subsequent needs of their children. The scope of work in perinatal substance abuse can include primary prevention, secondary prevention, and/or tertiary prevention.[1] Health care and human services personnel have contact with pregnant women who have not yet used alcohol and other drugs, with pregnant women who are currently using alcohol and other drugs, and with children and

From: *Drug and Alcohol Abuse Reviews, Vol. 8:*
Drug and Alcohol Abuse During Pregnancy and Childhood
Ed.: R. R. Watson ©1995 Humana Press Inc., Totowa, NJ

women who have suffered a negative impact of alcohol and other drug use. The number of women of childbearing age who use alcohol and other drugs and the number of drug-exposed infants have captured the attention of a variety of professions. These numbers have also focused the service and research dollars of federal and local agencies on the problems of substance-abusing pregnant and postpartum women and their children.

Perinatal substance abuse is an interdisciplinary concern. Like any complex human problem, the detection and treatment of perinatal substance abuse and its sequelae require the cooperation of a variety of health care and social service professionals. A woman who tests positive for drugs at labor and delivery will require the services of obstetricians, neonatologists, pediatricians, nurses, social workers, child welfare professionals, and substance abuse treatment experts within the first weeks of the child's life and, often, will continue to need a constellation of health and human services throughout her recovery and the child's development.

The attitudes, knowledge, and skills each professional brings to the treatment of a substance-abusing woman are the result of a combination of professional training and professional and personal experience. For many physicians, substance abuse is not a familiar area and may not have been part of formal medical training or residency training.[2] Nurses and social workers may have been exposed to basic levels of information about substance abuse screening and assessment techniques, but often are not familiar with referral mechanisms and substance abuse treatment issues salient for women. Child welfare professionals are just beginning to understand the impact of substance abuse on their work and the need for training programs.[3] Substance abuse treatment professionals have training and experience in screening, assessment, and treatment of substance abuse, but often are ill prepared to deal with the overlay of prenatal, postpartum, and well-baby care needs of women in early recovery. Substance abuse professionals also are in need of information about parenting education and child abuse prevention and how to integrate those services into treatment programming. Most health and human service professionals, regardless of discipline, are in need of additional training in domestic violence detection, treatment, and prevention.

Harrison[4] wrote that drug addiction during pregnancy can be seen as the interface between science, emotion, and social policy. Training programs in perinatal substance abuse must address this interface by providing information about attitudes, knowledge, and skills in substance abuse and in perinatal substance abuse.

This chapter is organized into three main sections: attitudes, knowledge, and skills. Under each of these sections, substance abuse training issues, in general, and perinatal substance abuse issues, in particular, are discussed. There exists a sizable collection of training curricula[5] and resource material in substance abuse and a growing number of resources in perinatal substance abuse. Examples of training resources are presented throughout the chapter. Given the diversity of professions involved in perinatal substance abuse and the variety of settings in which these professionals practice, it is unlikely that one training program will fill all professional and personal needs. The most effective training programs are most likely to be those that develop a list of their training needs in light of their services and populations. However, the issues addressed can reasonably apply to most professional staffs and settings.

Attitudes

Attitudes About Substance Abuse

An honest examination of attitudes is especially important in developing training in substance abuse; it is an area about which few people are neutral. Clark,[6] in his widely cited 1981 article, includes attitude as one of the four barriers to diagnosis and treatment of alcoholism. According to Clark, physicians who hold negative attitudes about people who abuse alcohol and/or who have a dim view of alcohol treatment efforts, will be less likely to diagnose alcohol problems than physicians who are more affirmative in their views. Although Clark wrote exclusively about physicians and alcoholism, his comments could be expanded to include other professionals and other drug abuse.

One of the familiar controversies in the alcohol and other drug literature is the debate over the disease concept of alcohol and other drug abuse. Is alcohol and other drug abuse a bad habit[7] or a disease?[8] Although many professional organizations have accepted the disease concept, not all individuals within those professions hold attitudes consonant with the idea that alcohol and other drug abuse is a chronic, relapsing illness that is influenced by genetic, environmental, and social influences. Deitch and Carleton[9] used the term "bias" to describe beliefs and attitudes that can affect treatment and training efforts. They described basic ideas about alcohol and other drug abuse that can generate controversies within staff groups. These areas include:

1. The disease process as the organizing concept for all drug dependence;
2. The benefits of working with an actively using person;
3. Definition of denial;
4. Variety and effectiveness of various treatment approaches;
5. Etiology; and
6. Abstinence as the cornerstone for recovery.

Several authors have presented models of alcohol abuse as a heuristic device to elicit attitudes about definition, etiology, and treatment. Rodgers and McMillin's[10] models varied on the etiology of the problem and the motivation of the individual who is struggling with it. The Family Welfare Research Group[11] included a section on models of drug abuse as a trigger for discussion in their skill-building curriculum for families with HIV and drug-affected children. Miller and Hester[12] presented 11 conceptual models of alcoholism and provided a discussion of each model's implications for intervention, thus showing that one's definition of the problem and its cause has clear impact on the action to remedy it.

Cultural beliefs regarding alcohol and other drug use are aspects of attitude exploration. The Institute on Black Chemical Abuse (IBCA)[13] developed a series of training programs and resource guides to examine cultural differences and culturally competent practices. The job of substance abuse training is to make explicit the implicit assumptions people hold about substance abuse and substance-abusing individuals. The goal of presenting competing explanatory models is not to force consensus or to develop a group orthodoxy, but to provide a level playing field for discussion and examination of attitudes important to setting and meeting treatment goals.

Attitudes About Perinatal Substance Abuse

A number of authors have written about the societal stigma substance-abusing women and mothers face.[14–16] Robbins[15] discussed stigma concerning women in sociological terms—stigma toward substance-abusing women is magnified because society sees substance-abusing women as deviating from socially sanctioned female roles. Substance-abusing women are seen as unable or unwilling to fend off unwanted sexual advances, and perhaps likely to initiate sexual activity. Blume[16] argued that the high rates of physical and sexual aggression among women who drink alcohol represent victimization rather than deviancy. Rates of childhood sexual abuse are also higher among drinking women. The media's portrayal of the relationship between cocaine abuse and sexual promiscuity among women contributes to the stigma associated with women who use substances.

Another area of stigma concerns the perception that substance-abusing women are seen as unable to fulfill maternal, child caring duties. It cannot be denied that maternal substance abuse plays a role in child abuse and neglect. Health care providers, especially those who work with drug-exposed, premature infants and/or with drug-exposed children with medical and learning problems, can hold negative attitudes toward the mothers. The titles of two recent videotapes concerning perinatal substance abuse, *Drug Babies*[17] and *Victims at Birth,*[18] indicate a perception that mothers victimize their children by using alcohol and drugs during pregnancy. *Victims at Birth* provides a view of a foster mother's anger toward a birth mother because of her polydrug abuse during pregnancy. Despite the titles, both these films present both the children and their substance-abusing mothers as victims in need of assistance and information, and are useful training resources.

The material published by the Women's Alcoholism Program of the Coalition on Addiction, Pregnancy, and Parenting (CASPAR)[19] includes several exercises to help people examine their feelings about alcoholic women. One of the training activities involves the generation of a list of statements commonly overheard about alcoholic women. The fact that most substance users are polysubstance abusers would warrant the inclusion of other drugs in such a discussion. The group is asked to list the images elicited by these statements. Participants are then asked to react to these statements as an alcoholic (or other drug abuser). The final step is to discuss the barriers these statements, images, and stereotypes create for women seeking and/or entering treatment.

This exercise is valuable because it requires participants to put themselves into the place of the alcoholic and other drug-abusing woman and to translate personal reactions into service barriers. A variation of this exercise is the "I am an alcoholic woman" activity. This activity asks each participant to read a prepared sentence that describes an alcoholic woman and her life circumstances. For example, "I am an alcoholic woman and my kid has no friends. I know it's my fault." While reading the sentence, the participant is instructed to think about a person he or she knows. A list of discussion questions follows to allow the group to express their feelings about the statements, the problems presented, the characteristics of the person, and the importance of the information and the feelings for treatment. This exercise personalizes the problems of alcoholic and other drug-abusing women and confronts stereotypes. The list prepared by the CASPAR group includes three statements specific to pregnant and postpartum women and 12 statements specific to motherhood. However, a knowledgeable group leader should be able to generate additional statements specific to the issues of perinatal substance abuse. By the same token, similar exercises can be constructed to elicit attitudes staff hold about child abuse, sexual victimization, and other comorbidity issues that affect women.

Videotape is another excellent avenue to engage people in discussions about their own attitudes as well as to expose them to the attitudes of substance-abusing women about their problems and their treatment. A recent release, entitled *Straight from the Heart: Stories of Mothers in Recovery,*[20] introduces six women, each of whom tells her own story of addiction, recovery, and parenthood. One of the compelling aspects of this tape is that the women talk about themselves as children, as wives and partners, as mothers, as alcoholics and other drug abusers, and as women in recovery. The discussion of competing roles can be useful in understanding the conflicts women face in trying to fulfill the demands of treatment and recovery as well as to provide care to their children.

The Attitudes About Drug Abuse in Pregnancy Question-naire is a more systematized attempt to evaluate attitudes.[21] Developed by Claire Coles, the questionnaire measures general knowledge about addiction and specific knowledge about prenatal exposure. In its current form, the questionnaire includes 54 statements about the effects of prenatal substance exposure, addiction, and its effects. The attitudes measured include punitive vs therapeutic, individual vs social responsibility, and negative vs positive stereotypes. The Attitudes About Drug Abuse in Pregnancy Questionnaire is in development and currently undergoing evaluation of content validity. This measure promises to be a useful tool for future research and training efforts in the area of perinatal substance abuse.

Although substance abuse is present among all socioeconomic groups, it is a special problem for low-income women. A comprehensive discussion of attitudes toward substance-abusing pregnant women will elicit attitudes toward poverty and racism. It is important that practitioners understand their clients' values and the cultural contexts of those values. For example, practitioners working with low-income substance-abusing teenagers need to understand gang values and to be able to interpret behaviors from the perspective of a gang member in addition to their personal and professional perspectives.

Knowledge
Knowledge About Substance Abuse

The attitudes held about a subject and the level of knowledge held about a subject are closely intertwined. Knowledge informs attitude and attitude invites additional knowledge. Practically speaking, training efforts often deal simultaneously with knowledge and attitudes, countering stereotypical images and mythology with facts and figures about alcohol and other drug use. As mentioned earlier, a number of training programs and curricula have been developed in the area of substance abuse. Knowledge-building programs on substance abuse typically include the following areas of information:

1. Definition of alcoholism and other drug abuse;
2. Biological, psychological, and social perspectives of alcohol and other drug abuse;
3. Signs and symptoms of alcohol and other drug abuse;
4. Denial; and
5. Information on the stages and progression of abuse.

Most training efforts have dealt primarily with alcoholism and, like the majority of research efforts, have been based on the needs of men. There is, however, a growing body of knowledge about women's experiences with alcohol and other drug abuse.

A useful overview of gender differences is offered by Lex,[22] who highlighted the salient issues from 20 yr of research on alcohol and other drug abuse. The consistent finding of the coexistence of sexual abuse and substance abuse among women is one area of attention. Root,[23] in an earlier work, discussed the failure of substance abuse professionals to address sexual victimization issues. Her view is that the omission of treatment for sexual victimization is a predominant reason women do not seek and/or complete substance abuse treatment programs. Harrison and Belille,[24] in a large sample of Midwestern treatment settings, highlighted the differences among women in treatment and noted that women younger than 30 were more likely to be polysubstance abusers, to have more mental health problems, and to have fewer social resources than women age 31 or older. One issue that should be emphasized in any training effort is that a percentage of women of childbearing age will use alcohol and/or other drugs during pregnancy, regardless of education, socioeconomic level, or ethnic identity. Mondanaro[25] wrote a textbook on the assessment and treatment of substance-abusing women that offers a sound overview of substance abuse issues, including information on cocaine and benzodiazepine dependency as well as about alcohol abuse. She included chapters on AIDS prevention, other coexisting conditions in substance-abusing women, and pregnancy and parenting. Although the topics are comprehensive, the volume is short enough to be useful in a time-limited training format. Another useful, shorter, and more recent overview of substance abuse among women is provided by Pape.[26] Wilsnack and Wilsnack's[27] panel study of the epidemiology of women's drinking is the gold standard in terms of understanding patterns, changes, and correlates of drinking behaviors among women. The CASPAR group provides one of the few training manuals that has been developed exclusively for professionals who work with women.[19] The manual includes information, handouts, and exercises for use with staff and client groups. Several knowledge-building exercises focus specifically on substance-abusing women and gender differences in use and consequences. Two sessions in this manual are devoted to facts and feelings about the use of alcohol and one session is devoted to prescription drug abuse among women.

The CASPAR group has also published a guide to detoxification of alcohol and other drug dependent, pregnant women.[28] This guide is especially helpful to health care professionals who are interested in developing links between substance abuse treatment and obstetrical and medical care. The detoxification guide includes articles on providing prenatal care to women with alcohol and drug problems.

An additional source of information about the facts and figures pertaining to women's use of alcohol and other drugs is the Center for Substance Abuse Prevention (CSAP). The *Prevention Resource Guide WOMEN,* as an example, is a short publication that is issued periodically and includes updated statistical information and descriptions of resource materials.[29]

CSAP's National Clearinghouse for Alcohol and Drug Information (1-800-729-6686) is a telephone service that is a good starting point for training programs looking for materials pertaining to substance abuse training.

Denial is a concept familiar to substance abuse professionals—one that deserves separate mention in relationship to women. Denial is the term used to convey client ambivalence or resistance to accept the existence of problems related to alcohol and other drug use. Denial has been seen as a barrier to assessment, diagnosis, and treatment. At one time, practitioners were taught to confront denial vigorously. However, more recent work in the field has encouraged practitioners to look more closely at patterns and reasons for resistance and to try to incorporate the client's perspective in making the implicit issues of alcohol and drug use explicit. Amodeo and Liftik[30] referred to this stance as working through denial and emphasized the avoidance of power struggles with clients. In working with substance-abusing women, instances of denial are more likely to indicate shame and guilt rather than resistance to treatment. Women who are resistant to assuming a label of alcoholic or drug abuser may not be denying the presence of a problem or rejecting help. They may be protecting themselves from another layer of stigma associated with alcohol and drug abuse. From a feminist perspective, Kasl[31] criticized much of the literature and protocol of the 12-step groups because of the tendency to reinforce and generate stigma among women. Her recommendations on ways to change 12-step group literature and her reformation about recovery for women are useful resources for training efforts. Empowerment appears to be a more useful concept than denial for understanding women.

Professionals working in perinatal substance abuse should know the basic levels and options of treatment efforts. Levels of treatment include detoxification, primary rehabilitation, and secondary rehabilitation; options refer to settings and include inpatient, outpatient, halfway house, and aftercare.[32] Within the levels and options, programs employ a variety of treatment approaches that can include abstinence, education, individual counseling, group counseling, aversion therapy, self-help groups, 12-step groups, cognitive behavioral counseling, and family counseling. The types of approaches and their use in treatment programs are well described in a number of texts.[33–35] Several training manuals on three specific treatment approaches are available from the National Institute on Alcohol Abuse and Alcoholism.[36–38] These manuals were developed for Project MATCH, the federally sponsored, multisite trial of patient-treatment matching. The three treatment approaches are:

1. Motivational Enhancement Therapy;
2. Twelve-Step Facilitation Therapy; and
3. Cognitive-Behavioral Coping Skills Therapy.

These manuals were developed for clinical research programs, but they are comprehensive and contain material that could be adapted for training individuals interested in the core principles of each therapeutic approach.

Knowledge About Perinatal Substance Abuse

Over the past several years, knowledge about perinatal substance abuse has grown. For example, Sonderegger[39] edited a text on the research findings and clinical implications of perinatal substance abuse. Walsh-Sukys and Kliegman[40] included a chapter on the treatment of cocaine addiction during pregnancy in a volume of controversies in perinatal care. O'Grady[41] included a chapter on perinatal substance abuse in an edited text of psychological and psychiatric syndromes in obstetrics. CSAP developed a resource guide for pregnant and postpartum women and their infants,[42] as well as the National

Perinatal Resource Center to provide a focus for knowledge development and training in the field of perinatal substance abuse. Interested readers can contact the Center through the National Clearinghouse.

One area of knowledge important to the topic of perinatal substance abuse is the effect of different substances and the combination of substances on the developing fetus. The level and technical specificity of this area of knowledge will, of course, differ with the audience. Physicians and nurses, for example, will most likely want more detailed information on teratogenic effects than other health professionals. Of importance, however, is that all professionals have an understanding of the reasons drug abuse during pregnancy is harmful so they can effectively explain why women should not use various drugs during pregnancy. Equally important is the need to understand the effects of drug exposure on the normal development of children to be able to screen for developmental delays and problems among growing children.

Knowledge about the dynamics of substance-abusing families is of particular importance in perinatal substance abuse. Research has demonstrated that alcoholism travels in families. It is likely to expect that some proportion of women who abuse alcohol and other drugs as adults grew up with parents who abused substances. This information on heredity has important implications for parenting issues and parent education efforts. Parent training efforts with substance-abusing women need to incorporate the fact that many substance-abusing women do not have role models for caring, nurturing parent–child relationships. Parent training curricula that nurture the parent as well as provide information and skill building are seen as preferable for use with substance-abusing women. Mothers in early recovery, who have few coping mechanisms other than alcohol and other drugs, can be at risk for relapse if they are not given additional resources to manage and understand behaviors of young children. Jesse[43] presented knowledge about substance-abusing families and offered a treatment model for healing parent–child relationships in these families.

Knowledge building can occur through a variety of activities. Classroom sessions, speakers, and discussion groups are among the most common training activities. Journal clubs, which meet weekly to discuss an article or a book chapter, are good ways to keep the area of perinatal substance abuse on the minds of the staff. Journal clubs are also excellent methods for keeping up to date with emerging information in the field. Case presentation and case staffing meetings can provide excellent teaching opportunities for the clinician prepared to lead a discussion of the substance abuse issues salient in the case. Case presentations can be especially effective in multidisciplinary settings where staff have varying levels of interest and expertise in substance abuse.

Skills

Screening in Perinatal Substance Abuse

All personnel working with women and working with pregnant and postpartum women should be able to conduct a basic screening interview to identify women at risk for substance abuse. Screening efforts are different from assessment efforts, which are more detailed and comprehensive. Many screening tools have been developed for use with people who abuse alcohol. The CAGE questionnaire[44] and the HEAT questionnaire[45] are familiar screening tools, which receive their names using the acronym from each of the four screening questions that comprise them. Both the CAGE and the HEAT are broad screening tools for use in the general population, but the HEAT is preferable because it asks questions that encourage discussion of patterns of use and includes the opportunity to discuss reasons for use and to talk about relationships with other people. The questions in the HEAT tool are:

1. *How* do you use alcohol?
2. Have you ever thought you used to *excess?*
3. Has *anyone* else ever thought you used too much? and
4. Have you ever had any *trouble* resulting from your use?

A positive response to questions 2, 3, or 4 in the HEAT indicates a risk of alcohol abuse and warrants a fuller, more formal assessment. Although the HEAT is simple and easy to use, it is not specific about the time of the alcohol use or the trouble associated with it. This lack of time frame is also true of the CAGE. Jacobson[46] suggested a simple addition, a question asking "When?" in response to any affirmative answer. Another obvious limitation is that the HEAT, as written, focuses solely on alcohol use, but a simple addition of a phrase such as "alcohol, cocaine, or other drugs" in the first question remedies that limitation. Standardized screening tests include the Michigan Alcoholism Screening Test (MAST)[47] and the Drug Abuse Screening Test (DAST),[48] both of which have shortened forms. They are easy to administer and can provide a set of discussion items as well as a score indicating problems with alcohol and other drugs. Russell[49] presented an excellent review article on new assessment tools for risk drinking during pregnancy.

Using a list of risk factors is another screening technique. Miller and Doucette[50] developed a list of behavioral indicators for substance abuse during pregnancy. These indicators include:

1. Admission of use of alcohol and other drugs prior to pregnancy;
2. Lack of prenatal care;
3. Entering prenatal care late in pregnancy;
4. Sporadic prenatal care;

5. Premature labor, premature delivery, or abruptio placentae; and/or
6. Stillbirth or birth of an infant with anomalies.

These behavioral indicators in combination with a set of screening questions can provide adequate evidence for a practitioner to move on to a more comprehensive assessment process. Miller and Doucette offered a list of recommended baseline questions that could be incorporated into a medical history protocol and used with all women seeking care. Tocco et al.[51] offered recommendations on practical diagnostic and counseling guidelines for clinicians working with substance-abusing pregnant women.

Assessment in Perinatal Substance Abuse

All personnel working in health and human service settings with women need to be able to recognize the signs and symptoms of alcohol and drug abuse and to complete a brief screening interview. Not all personnel need to be trained in comprehensive assessment and diagnostic techniques. Assessment techniques include the use of standardized interview protocols, personal interviews, and, in some circumstances, toxicology screening and medical examinations. The outcome of assessment is diagnosis and treatment, and only those women who have some indication of the presence of alcohol and other drug abuse should receive a full assessment. Standardized assessment instruments include the Addiction Severity Index (ASI),[52] a 180-item test that is completed by a trained interviewer during a 30–45 min session. The Maternal Post Partum Interview was developed to collect information about alcohol and other drug use during pregnancy.[53] This instrument also requires a trained interviewer to administer it.

Some professionals are less interested in standardized instruments and prefer to use an assessment interview to gather information about alcohol and other drug use. The CASPAR manual, *Getting Sober, Getting Well*,[19] offers a sample of an alcohol intake form and an intake form for prescribed and over-the-counter medicines. Lewis et al.[34] also provided a sample psychosocial and substance abuse history instrument, a sample behavioral assessment and functional analysis instrument, and a sample comprehensive drinker profile. General areas of questions in an assessment form should include frequency, quantity, and pattern of use for all substances. Inclusion of tobacco as an addictive substance is important for all people, but especially important for pregnant women because of the association of maternal smoking with poor birth outcomes. Other areas to include: concerns the patient has about substance use, the consequences the client associates with substance use, and any history of treatment or attempts to quit. Information about sexual victimization, either current or past, is essential in assessing women's use of alcohol and other drugs. Worell and Remer[54] presented an excellent chapter on confronting abuse that offers a scale of attitudes about abusive relationships, research findings, strategies for intervention, and training exercises.

Motivational Interviewing

Knowledge on how to use screening and assessment tools is necessary, but not sufficient for effective practice with substance-abusing women. Clinicians who are not able to engage their patients in a process of change may gather a lot of information, but can expect relatively poor outcomes in terms of entry into treatment, compliance with treatment protocols, and decreased substance use. Pregnancy presents a clinical opportunity for change and many pregnant women are looking for ways to quit using alcohol and other drugs, but are unsure how to seek help without risking punishment and stigma.

Motivational interviewing is the term Miller and Rollnick gave to their efforts to help clients decide to make changes in their lives.[36,55] The conceptual background for motivational interviewing lies in the work of Prochaska and DiClemente,[56] who stated that all changed behavior can be discussed in terms of six stages:

1. Precontemplation;
2. Contemplation;
3. Determination;
4. Action;
5. Maintenance; and
6. Relapse.

Stages 2–6 are arranged graphically in circular form and represent "different stages of readiness for change" (as cited in Miller and Rollnick[55]). The professional's job is to help the client recognize his or her readiness for change and to provide motivation for him or her to move to the next stage of change. The approach relies on a nondirective approach that emphasizes strengths and minimizes confrontation, argument, and authoritarian stances. In a controlled comparison of therapist style, motivational interviewing techniques were associated with less client resistance, which was associated with better outcomes after 1 yr.[57] Chapter 5 of the Miller and Rollnick volume presents the principles of motivational interviewing and contrasts these principles with traditional counseling techniques. The information in this chapter could easily be adapted to a training format and used to train personnel. Training curricula and videotaped sessions on motivational interviewing are also available.

Life Skills Training
for Women Who Abuse Alcohol and Other Drugs

IBCA has made the distinction between habilitation and rehabilitation and living skills and survival skills.[58] Habilitation is defined as the establishment of the most common cultural norms of social living and rehabilitation is the reestablishment of those norms. Many women who abuse substances during pregnancy require habilitation in developing healthy social behaviors. Just as women need to change their alcohol and drug use patterns, they need to change their social behaviors and their expectations of themselves and others. Comprehensive programming for substance-abusing pregnant women needs to continue well after screening, assessment, and treatment to provide basic life skills training, such as budgeting, manners, job seeking skills, vocational training, and parenting education. Development of these long-term skills is essential to support long-term recovery for both mothers and children.

References

[1] L. D. Gilchrist and M. R. Gillmore (1992) Methodological issues in prevention research on drug use and pregnancy, in *Methodological Issues in Epidemiological, Prevention, and Treatment Research on Drug-Exposed Women and Their Children.* M. M. Kilbey and K. Asghar, eds. Research Monograph 117, National Institute on Drug Abuse, US Department of Health and Human Services, Rockville, MD, pp. 1–17.

[2] J. N. Chappel and D. C. Lewis (1992) Medical education in substance abuse, in *Substance Abuse: A Comprehensive Textbook,* 2nd Ed. J. Lowinson, P. Ruiz, and R. Millman, eds. Williams and Wilkins, Baltimore, MD, pp. 958–969.

[3] E. M. Tracy and K. J. Farkas (1994) Preparing practitioners for child welfare practice with substance abusing families. *Child Welfare* **73(1),** 57–68.

[4] M. Harrison (1991) Drug addiction in pregnancy: the interface of science, emotion, and social policy. *J. Subst. Abuse Treatment* **8,** 261–268.

[5] A. K. Davis, T. V. Parran, and A. V. Graham (1993) Educational strategies for clinicians. *Primary Care* **29,** 241–250.

[6] W. D. Clark (1981) Blocks to diagnosis and treatment. *Am. J. Med.* **71,** 275–286.

[7] H. Fingarette (1991) We should reject the disease concept of alcoholism. *Harvard Med. Sch. Mental Health Lett.* **6,** 4.

[8]G. Valliant (1990) We should retain the disease concept of alcoholism. *Harvard Med. Sch. Mental Health Lett.* **6,** 4.

[9]D. A. Deitch and S. A. Carleton (1992) Education and training of clinical personnel, in *Substance Abuse: A Comprehensive Textbook,* 2nd Ed. J. Lowinson, P. Ruiz, and R. Millman, eds. Williams and Wilkins, Baltimore, MD, pp. 970–982.

[10]R. L. Rodgers and C. S. McMillin (1988) *Don't Help: A Guide to Working with the Alcoholic.* Madrona Press, Seattle, WA.

[11]Family Welfare Research Group (1992) *Family Power: Building Skills for Families with HIV and Drug-Affected Children.* University of California at Berkeley, Berkeley, CA.

[12]W. R. Miller and R. K. Hester (1989) Treating alcohol problems: toward an informed eclecticism, in *Handbook of Alcoholism Treatment Approaches: Effective Alternatives.* R. K. Hester and W. R. Miller, eds. Pergamon, New York, pp. 3–13.

[13]Institute on Black Chemical Abuse (1990) *Developing Chemical Dependency Services for Black People.* Author, Minneapolis, MN.

[14]W. H. George, S. J. Gournic, and M. P. McAfee (1988) Perceptions of post drinking female sexuality: effects of gender, beverage choice, and drink payment. *J. Appl. Soc. Psychol.* **18,** 1295–1317.

[15]C. Robbins (1989) Sex differences in psychosocial consequences of alcohol and drug abuse. *J. Health Soc. Behav.* **30,** 117–130.

[16]S. Blume (1991) Sexuality and stigma: the alcoholic woman. *Alcohol Health Res. World* **15,** 139–146.

[17]Y. Parsons, Producer (1990) *Drug Babies* (videotape). Parsons Runyon Arts and Entertainment, Santa Barbara, CA.

[18]*Victims at Birth* (videotape). (1990) University of California Extension Media Center, Berkeley, CA.

[19]N. Finkelstein, S. A. Duncan, L. Derman, and J. Smeltz (1990) *Getting Sober, Getting Well: A Treatment Guide for Caregivers Who Work with Women.* The Women's Alcoholism Program of the Coalition on Addiction, Pregnancy, and Parenting, Cambridge, MA.

[20]*Straight from the Heart: Stories of Mothers Recovering from Addiction* (videotape) (1991) Vida Health Productions and NAACOG, Cambridge, MA.

[21]C. Coles (1990) *The Attitudes About Drug Abuse Questionnaire.* Emory University, Atlanta, GA.

[22]B. W. Lex (1991) Some gender differences in alcohol and polysubstance users. *Health Psychol.* **10,** 121–132.

[23]M. M. P. Root (1989) Treatment failures: the role of sexual victimization in women's addictive behavior. *Am. J. Orthopsychiat.* **59,** 542–549.

[24]P. A. Harrison and C. A. Belille (1987) Women in treatment: beyond the stereotype. *J. Stud. Alcohol* **28,** 574–578.

[25]J. Mondanaro (1989) *Chemically Dependent Women: Assessment and Treatment.* Lexington Books, Lexington, MA.

[26]P. A. Pape (1993) Issues in assessment and intervention with alcohol and drug-abusing women, in *Clinical Work with Substance-Abusing Clients.* S. L. A. Straussner, ed. Guilford, New York, pp. 251–296.

[27]S. C. Wilsnack and R. W. Wilsnack (1991) Epidemiology of women's drinking. *J. Subst. Abuse* **3,** 133–157.

[28]Coalition on Addiction, Pregnancy, and Parenting (undated) *A Guide to the Detoxification of Alcohol and Other Drug Dependent, Pregnant Women.* Author, Cambridge, MA.

[29]Center for Substance Abuse Prevention (October, 1991) *Prevention Resource Guide WOMEN.* Public Health Service, Substance Abuse and Mental Health Services Administration, ADM-91-187, US Department of Health and Human Services, Rockville, MD.

[30]M. Amodeo and J. Liftik (1990) Working through denial in alcoholism. *J. Contemp. Hum. Serv.* **71,** 131–135.

[31]C. D. Kasl (1992) *Many Roads, One Journey, Moving Beyond the Twelve Steps.* Harper Perennial, New York.

[32]K. J. Farkas and T. V. Parran (1993) Treatment of cocaine addiction during pregnancy, in *Current Controversies in Perinatal Care II. Clinics in Perinatology,* 20,1. M. C. Walsh-Sukys and R. M. Kliegman, eds. Saunders, Philadelphia, pp. 29–45.

[33]R. K. Hester and W. R. Miller (eds.) (1989) *Handbook of Alcoholism Treatment Approaches: Effective Alternatives.* Pergamon, New York.

[34]J. A. Lewis, R. Q. Dana, and G. A. Blevins (1994) *Substance Abuse Counseling: An Individualized Approach,* 2nd Ed. Brooks-Cole, Pacific Grove, CA.

[35]S. L. A. Straussner (ed.) (1993) *Clinical Work with Substance-Abusing Clients.* Guilford, New York.

[36]National Institute on Alcohol Abuse and Alcoholism (1992) *Motivational Enhancement Therapy Manual: A Clinical Research Guide for Therapists Treating Individuals with Alcohol Abuse and Dependence.* Public Health Service, Alcohol, Drug Abuse, and Mental Health

Administration, National Institute on Alcohol Abuse and Alcoholism, US Department of Health and Human Services, US Government Printing Office, 331-126/70214, Washington, DC.

[37]National Institute on Alcohol Abuse and Alcoholism (1992) *Twelve Step Facilitation Therapy Manual: A Clinical Research Guide for Therapists Treating Individuals with Alcohol Abuse and Dependence.* Public Health Service, Alcohol, Drug Abuse, and Mental Health Administration, US Department of Health and Human Services, US Government Printing Office, 331-128/70215, Washington, DC.

[38]National Institute on Alcohol Abuse and Alcoholism (1992) *Cognitive-Behavioral Coping Skills Therapy Manual: A Clinical Research Guide for Therapists Treating Individuals with Alcohol Abuse and Dependence.* Public Health Service, Alcohol, Drug Abuse, and Mental Health Administration, US Department of Health and Human Services, US Government Printing Office, 331-127/70216, Washington, DC.

[39]T. B. Sonderegger (ed.) (1992) *Perinatal Substance Abuse: Research Findings and Clinical Implications.* Johns Hopkins University Press, Baltimore, MD.

[40]M. C. Walsh-Sukys and R. M. Kliegman (eds.) (1993) *Current Controversies in Perinatal Care II. Clinics in Perinatology.* Saunders, Philadelphia.

[41]J. P. O'Grady (ed.) (1992) *Obstetrics: Psychological and Psychiatric Syndromes.* Elsevier, New York.

[42]Center for Substance Abuse Prevention (1991) *Prevention Resource Guide: Pregnant/Postpartum Women and Their Infants.* Public Health Service, Substance Abuse and Mental Health Services Administration, US Department of Health and Human Services, ADM-91-1804, Rockville, MD.

[43]R. C. Jesse (1989) *Children in Recovery.* Norton, New York.

[44]D. Mayfield, G. McLeod, and P. Hall (1974) The CAGE questionnaire: validation of a new alcoholism screening instrument. *Am. J. Psychiatry* **131,** 1121–1123.

[45]M. Willinbring (1988) Evaluating alcohol use in elders. *Generations* **12,** 27–31.

[46]G. R. Jacobson (1989) A comprehensive approach to pretreatment evaluation: I. Detection, assessment and diagnosis of alcoholism, in *Handbook of Alcoholism Treatment Approaches: Effective Alternatives.* R. K. Hester and W. R. Miller, eds. Pergamon, New York, pp. 17–53.

[47]M. L. Selzer (1971) The Michigan Alcoholism Screening Test: the quest for a new diagnostic instrument. *Am. J. Psychiatry* **127,** 29.

[48]H. Skinner (1982) The Drug Abuse Screening Test. *Addict. Behav.* **7,** 363–371.

[49]M. Russell (1994) New assessment tools for risk drinking during pregnancy: T-ACE, TWEAK, and others. *Alcohol Health Res. World* **18,** 55–61.

[50]W. H. Miller and M. G. Doucette (1992) Perinatal substance abuse, in *Obstetrics: Psychological and Psychiatric Syndromes.* J. P. O'Grady, ed. Elsevier, New York, pp. 163–179.

[51]R. V. Tocco, R. F. Klein, and M. Friedman-Campbell (1993) History taking and substance abuse counseling with the pregnant patient. *Clin. Obstet. Gynecol.* **36,** 338–346.

[52]A. T. McLellan, L. Luborsky, G. E. Woody, and C. P. O'Brien (1980) An improved diagnostic evaluation instrument for substance abuse patients: the Addiction Severity Index. *J. Nerv. Ment. Disord.* **168,** 26.

[53]A. P. Streissguth (1986) Smoking and drinking during pregnancy and offspring learning disabilities, in *Learning Disabilities and Prenatal Risk.* M. Lewis, ed. University of Illinois Press, Urbana-Champaign, IL, pp. 28–39.

[54]J. Worell and P. Remer (1992) *Feminist Perspectives in Therapy: An Empowerment Model for Women.* Wiley, New York.

[55]W. R. Miller and S. Rollnick (1991) *Motivational Interviewing: Preparing People to Change Addictive Behavior.* Guilford, New York.

[56]J. O. Prochaska and C. C. DiClemente (1986) Toward a comprehensive model of change, in *Handbook of Alcoholism Treatment Approaches: Effective Alternatives.* R. K. Hester and W. R. Miller, eds. Pergamon, New York, pp. 3–27.

[57]W. R. Miller, R. G. Benefield, and J. Scott Tonigan (1993) Enhancing motivation for change in problem drinking: a controlled comparison of two therapist styles. *J. Consult. Clin. Psychol.* **61,** 455–461.

[58]Institute on Black Chemical Abuse (1992) *Overview of Cultural Sensitivity and Specificity.* Author, Minneapolis, MN.

Psychosocial Factors Affecting Rural Adolescent Alcohol Use

Tami J. Hedges, Meg Gerrard, Frederick X. Gibbons, and Gabie E. Smith

Introduction

Driving while under the influence of alcohol, being involved in automobile accidents, and engaging in precocious and/or unprotected sexual intercourse are some of the myriad of problems associated with adolescent alcohol consumption. In the past, such problems were considered to be primarily an urban phenomenon.[1] Over the past decade, however, ample evidence has shown that these problems have spread to rural America. For example, between 1982 and 1988 the number of 15–24 yr olds in Iowa dropped from 260,000 to 201,000, but the number of fatal motor vehicle accidents involving adolescents remained stable. The result was a 23% increase in the proportion of young drivers who were involved in fatal

From: *Drug and Alcohol Abuse Reviews, Vol. 8:*
Drug and Alcohol Abuse During Pregnancy and Childhood
Ed.: R. R. Watson ©1995 Humana Press Inc., Totowa, NJ

accidents.[2] There has been a similar increase in the rate of teenage pregnancies. In 1980, the rate of teen out-of-wedlock births in Iowa ranked 49th among the 50 states, but by 1990 25% of the births in Iowa were out-of-wedlock, bringing Iowa up to the median of the country.[3,4] The myth of problem-free rural life in contrast with the volatility of urban problems continues, however, and has contributed to the relative paucity of research on the antecedents of rural adolescents' behavior problems, such as alcohol use.

The general purpose of this chapter is to review the research on social-psychological factors related to adolescent alcohol use, especially as it occurs in rural settings. The specific purposes of this chapter are threefold: First, to document the prevalence of adolescent alcohol consumption in general, and among rural adolescents in particular; second, to review previous studies investigating the antecedents of rural adolescent alcohol use; and third, to report findings from our own prospective investigations of factors associated with adolescent alcohol use in rural America.

Prevalence of Alcohol Use Among Rural Adolescents

Adolescence has often been viewed as a time of experimentation with a variety of potentially dangerous behaviors (e.g., "risky" sex, reckless driving, substance abuse).[5,6] Foremost among these, at least in terms of prevalence, is alcohol consumption. One study involving a national sample of over 100,000 adolescents reported that 77% of 8th graders had tried alcohol at some time; by the 12th grade, 93% of the sample reported having at least tried alcohol.[7] Another study of adolescents in Los Angeles found that 98.6% of these students had tried alcohol. Even more surprising, 93.8% reported that they used alcohol monthly.[8] Likewise, a sample of San Francisco East Bay 14 yr olds reported that 5% used alcohol frequently, 45% said they used alcohol in various amounts, and another 45% had at least tried alcohol.[9] Remarkably, these results indicate that only 5% of urban 14 yr olds had *not* tried alcohol.

As we noted, most of the studies in this area have focused on alcohol prevalence among urban youth. Partly because of the farm crisis of the 1980s, however, research is now beginning to focus on rural adolescents' risky behaviors. One such study of 8th and 10th graders in Texas found that rural communities near metropolitan areas were certainly not immune to the problems that plagued the neighboring cities; instead, these rural adolescents had violence and drug-use patterns that were similar to those of their urban counterparts.[10] Oetting and Beauvais[7] also found comparable alcohol use in rural and national samples: 91% of their rural high school seniors had used alcohol, whereas 93% of the national sample of this age had used alcohol.

Some studies have suggested that rural adolescents may even have alcohol use rates that exceed national averages for their cohort. For example, a study of rural Michigan middle school students found young rural adolescents had alcohol misuse rates well above the national average.[11] Similar results were found in rural Rocky Mountain areas, where between 91 and 93% of the 8th graders and 92–100% of the 12th graders reported trying alcohol. The mean for the Rocky Mountain Region seniors was 97%, which was significantly greater than the mean for the national sample of the same age.[12] A study of rural 7th, 8th, and 9th graders from Pennsylvania indicated that 62% of these students reported they had gotten drunk at least once, 20% at least once a month, and 16% at least once a week.[13] Finally, as can be seen in Table 1, the prevalence of alcohol use in rural Iowa adolescents and college students from our own prospective study is quite comparable to that reported in other studies of rural adolescents.

Table 1
Alcohol Use in Rural Iowa Adolescents
and Iowa College Freshmen[a]

| | Percentage of students responding | | | |
| | Adolescent sample[b] | | College sample[c] | |
Response	Time 1	Time 2	Time 1	Time 2
Never	72	57	23	11
Once or twice	13	16	18	10
A few times	10	17	27	30
More than a few times	3	8	22	29
Regularly	1	2	10	19

[a]Measure: "How many times in the last 3 months have you had a whole drink of alcohol?"

[b]The Adolescent Time 1 sample consisted of 500 8th and 10th graders, and the Time 2 sample consisted of the same students in the 9th and 11th grades (T2, $N = 476$).

[c]The College Time 1 sample consisted of 679 students at the beginning of their freshman year, and the Time 2 sample consisted of the same students after they had been in college for 6 mo (T2, $N = 628$).

In short, whether it is Texas, Michigan, Colorado, Pennsylvania, or Iowa, rural areas are not "safe havens" from alcohol use. Rural adolescents use alcohol at rates similar to, or perhaps even slightly above, national levels, and so there is every reason to believe that they are susceptible to all of the problems that affect urban adolescent drinkers.

Problems Associated with Alcohol Use

According to most researchers in the area, risk behaviors such as alcohol consumption do not occur in isolation. For example, Jessor and Jessor[14] postulated a Problem Behavior

Syndrome, which suggests that teenagers who engage in one risk behavior are very likely to engage in other problem behaviors. One such problem behavior, which often follows alcohol use, is drunk driving. Adolescents are exposed to alarmingly high levels of risk from automobile accidents, both from driving while under the influence of alcohol and from being passengers in cars driven by drunk drivers.[15] That point is made convincingly in a recent study involving nearly 7000 rural Mississippi students.[16] The percentage of these students who reported they had driven while under the influence of alcohol ranged from 5% in the 7th grade to 27% in the 12th grade. The percentage of students who said they had been a passenger in a car driven by a teenage driver under the influence of alcohol was even higher, ranging from 35% in the 7th grade to 46% in the 12th grade.

Another potentially dangerous behavior that has been shown to be closely associated with alcohol consumption is risky sexual behavior. Specifically, alcohol use has been found to correlate with earlier onset of initial sexual intercourse and with number of sexual partners. It is also associated with an increase in unprotected sexual intercourse.[17] For example, in a study of Massachusetts adolescents, 64% reported having had sex after drinking and 17% admitted that they used condoms less often after drinking than when they were not drinking.[18] An additional study involving 43 young women who had experienced an unplanned pregnancy found that 33% of the women reported they had been drinking when they got pregnant.[19]

There is no question that rural adolescents are using alcohol and that they are being exposed to the problems that come with adolescent drinking. It is also clear that for adolescents, alcohol use is primarily a social event. In fact, although young people drink significantly less often than adults, when they do drink, they drink more at any given time and are more likely than adults to do their drinking in social settings.[20] Thus, it is not surprising that a number of studies have shown a link between adolescent drinking and a variety of social influences and social cognitions.[21] The following sections summarize these social psychological antecedents of adolescent alcohol consumption.

Antecedents and Influences on Adolescent Alcohol Use

Social Influence: The Role of Social Settings, Peers, and Parents

The social influence approach to understanding adolescent alcohol use maintains that social settings, peers, and parents influence adolescent alcohol use through either modeling or normative pressure. The modeling literature, for example, has suggested that adolescents will learn to drink or not to drink after exposure to a drinker, usually a parent or friend.[22–24] Normative influence involves the social setting and the associated perceived standards of conduct. In the case of drinking, this approach would suggest that adolescents drink if they believe their drinking is approved of by other people (e.g., parents and friends) and if it is sanctioned by the situation (e.g., during social activities).[25]

Social Settings

Consistent with these hypotheses, a number of studies have revealed that the amount of time spent in extracurricular activities and church activities is negatively correlated with alcohol use. One example of this is early research by Hirschi,[26] which suggested that adolescents with high levels of involvement and commitment to either the family or structured activities (e.g., school and sports) were less likely to engage in risky behaviors, in general, including alcohol use. A recent study in rural Pennsylvania found that regular drinkers tended to receive lower grades in school, participate less in sponsored extracurricular activities, have worse family relations, and attend church less frequently.[13] In fact, religiosity has consistently been found to negatively correlate with alcohol use,[27] whereas frequency of attending religious services, in particular, is negatively associated with alcohol use among rural adolescents.[28]

Other studies have found that the amount of time spent in certain kinds of social activities (e.g., parties) was positively related to alcohol use.[28] Of course there is an obvious distinction between Bloch et al.'s definition of extracurricular activities and S. Gibbons et al.'s social situations. Whereas Bloch's extracurricular activities included supervised social activities, such as school sports and school clubs, S. Gibbons' social situations included unsponsored and unsupervised activities, such as "cruising" and parties. S. Gibbons et al.[28] suggested that parties act as a cue to drink primarily because of media attempts to convince young people that parties, good times, and alcohol are a necessary threesome. An additional study of rural Pennsylvania high school students found similar correlates with alcohol use—heavy alcohol users enjoyed school less, received lower grades, and participated in more unsupervised social activities.[29]

Peers

Social psychological theories, such as The Theory of Reasoned Action,[30,31] suggest that the decision to engage in a particular behavior, whether risky or not, is a function of two factors: perceived norms ("What would others think of this behavior?") and motivation to comply with these norms ("Do I care what others think?"). In fact, the desire to comply with perceived expectations of friends and peers has often been cited as the major reason why adolescents engage in certain risk behaviors.[32,33] For example, a study of 5th and 6th graders from urban Michigan schools found that frequency of alcohol use was related to the students' desire to comply with peer pressure.[34] It must be acknowledged, however, that peer influence and problem behaviors are related in a reciprocal manner. On the one hand, peers may encourage a variety of risk behaviors, such as alcohol use and sex;[35] on the other hand, people who wish to engage in these behaviors are also likely to seek out friends who engage in similar behaviors. For example, Conger et al.[36] found that rural Iowa adolescents with antisocial tendencies tend to seek out friends who are also antisocial. Thus, personality factors and peer influence interact to increase the frequency of problem behaviors.

Parental Influence

Not surprisingly, parents or guardians have also been shown to have a significant social influence on adolescent drinking behavior.[37] In addition to the obvious impact that parents have through modeling and normative influence, recent research has suggested that family conflict and hostility are also linked to adolescents' alcohol use. For example, in a longitudinal replication of Elder's[38] classic research on Depression-era families, Conger et al.[36] examined the influence of the "farm crisis" of the 1980s on adolescent alcohol use. Conger's findings revealed a "path way" of alcohol influence, which began with the impact that family economic pressure had on parental hostility. That hostility was then directed toward the children and, as a result, was linked to antisocial adolescent behavior. This behavior, in turn, was associated with seeking antisocial friends, and then, finally, with using alcohol. In short, these data do not support a direct link between parental behavior and adolescent drinking—rather, antisocial behavior and having antisocial friends mediate the relation between the parents' hostility and their children's alcohol use. It should be noted that this was a longitudinal study, and that it employed videotaped interactions between the parents and adolescents that were coded by independent raters. Thus, the data included raters' judgments of parents' expressions of hostility, in addition to the parents', adolescents', and siblings' impressions of the interactions. Because of this, the study makes a strong case for the influence of family dynamics on adolescent alcohol use. In addition, it has made an important contribution to the existing literature on social influence by demonstrating that parental and peer influence interact to influence adolescent alcohol use.

Personality Antecedents

No review of the literature on the antecedents of adolescent alcohol use would be complete without mention of individual differences. Unfortunately, much of the research that has investigated the role of personality variables on adolescent alcohol use has resulted in inconsistent findings. For example, some studies have found a relation between self-esteem and alcohol use, whereas others have not.[13,27,39] This inconsistency can be seen in a series of studies by Donovan and Jessor.[40] In one of their studies, these authors reported that self-esteem in early youth was negatively correlated with problem drinking among males, but positively correlated among females. In a second study reported in that article, the same researchers found that self-esteem in adolescence was uncorrelated with later problem drinking among males and females. These inconsistent results suggest that the relation between self-esteem and drinking is not simple, but rather involves other mediators or moderators that have not yet been adequately captured in the research.

There is one individual difference measure that has consistently been linked with adolescent drinking, however, and that is sensation seeking.[41] Adolescents who exhibit a general willingness to explore and experiment with new things also are likely to intend to drink in the future[42] and, eventually, are more likely to drink.[43,44]

Cognitive Influences
on Adolescent Alcohol Use

Recently, a number of social–cognitive factors have also been shown to predict the initiation of adolescent drinking. We now describe two closely related lines of research that explore the impact of these cognitive factors on teen drinking; these approaches involve expectancy theory and social images. This discussion is followed by an introduction to our own research regarding the influence of prototype perceptions on adolescent drinking.

Expectancy Theory

Alcohol-related expectancies have been defined as cognitive representations of a person's past experience with alcohol, as well as their perceptions of the costs and benefits associated with drinking.[45] That is, adolescents who have previously used alcohol will have future alcohol expectancies that match their past experience—if they had fun drinking at a party, for example, they will have positive alcohol expectancies. On the other hand, adolescents who have never used alcohol will have expectancies based on what they imagine would happen to them if they were to drink.[46] Thus, if an adolescent's friends were to tell him or her that drinking makes them sick, then it is likely the adolescent will have negative alcohol expectancies.

McLaughlin-Mann et al.[47] examined several alcohol expectancies, including: expectancies of altered social behavior (i.e., becoming more outgoing and more popular), altered cognitive and motor functioning (e.g., loss of reaction time), tension reduction (i.e., relaxation), and personal motives (e.g., changes in self-perceptions, such as seeing oneself as more favorable). As expected, these alcohol expectancies were found to be predictive of both current alcohol involvement and risk for future alcoholism.

Social Images

One type of expectancy associated with alcohol use is the image that adolescents believe is associated with a particular behavior.[48,49] Early research on this concept suggested that these images are related to the behavior itself. For example, research on the social images associated with smoking indicated that adolescents whose self-concepts were similar to their perception of the prototypical adolescent smoker were more likely to smoke.[50,51]

More recently, Chassin et al.[52] suggested that social images also influence alcohol use. They postulated the following reasons why images may be important in adolescent drinking. First, according to consistency theory, people are more likely to engage in a behavior if it is consistent with their self-concept. For example, an adolescent who has a self-concept that includes risk taking and adventure may believe the drinking image fits their self-image. Second, drinking can have some instrumental value, because it may make the adolescent acquire an image to which he or she may aspire.[53] For example, if adolescents believe that their friends have a positive image of a drinker—perhaps "cool" or independent—they may drink so their friends will view them in a positive way.[52]

Prototype Perception

The approach that we have taken in our research with adolescents is similar to that taken by these "image researchers" and is based on three primary assumptions. First, we assume that adolescent alcohol use, like all adolescent risk behaviors, is primarily a social phenomenon. These behaviors are performed in the presence of, and often for the benefit of, friends and peers. Second, we believe that adolescents, in general, possess an image or a representation of the type of person who drinks—a prototype of the typical adolescent drinker. Third, this prototype is related to willingness to drink.[54]

Consistent with this reasoning, the research that we have conducted has demonstrated that the more favorable the prototype of the typical adolescent drinker is and the more similar individuals think they are to the prototypical drinker, the more likely they are to drink.[35,55,56]

Conclusions from the Literature

To summarize, rural and urban adolescents have similar rates of alcohol use and drinking appears to be a social phenomenon for both groups. It is not surprising, then, that social influence and social cognitions have been identified as correlates of adolescent alcohol use. Much of the past research has been limited in a variety of aspects, however. Specifically, very few of the studies were longitudinal in design, making it impossible to understand the causal relations between these variables and the dynamic nature of alcohol use. In addition, previous studies have not comprehensively examined both social (family and peer) influence and cognitive factors. And finally, few studies have specifically focused on rural samples.

The Iowa Health and Behavior Research Project

In response to some of these limitations, we developed the Iowa Health and Behavior Risk Project to examine the influences of family, friends, and cognitive mediators (e.g., perceptions of prototypes) on health risk behaviors. In particular, this study is an ongoing longitudinal project to investigate four types of adolescent risk behavior: alcohol use; risky sexual behavior, including unprotected sex; reckless driving; and smoking. One primary hypothesis explored in this research is that prototype perceptions predict drinking among college students and adolescents. Specifically, the more favorable the perception is, and the more similar to the self it is thought to be, the more willing the adolescent will be to engage in the behavior. Both the similarity and the favorability components of the prototype perception are important. Similarity reflects the individual's identification with the prototype and the group it represents. Favorability indicates the attractiveness the behavior (e.g., drinking) and the group (e.g., drinkers) have for the individual. Using alcohol as an example, the specific prediction is that college students and adolescents who have favorable perceptions of the "typical" drinker their age, and who believe they are similar to that prototype, will drink more than those who view the prototype negatively.

Two different samples are being used in this project. The first consists of 679 college freshman at Iowa State University from rural and urban areas in Iowa, and the second includes 500 adolescents attending public schools in rural Iowa. The parents of both samples also participated in the study. (More complete descriptions of the samples can be found in F. X. Gibbons et al.[56,57])

College Sample

Participants in the college sample completed the initial questionnaire (Time 1) within the first 2 wk of their arrival on campus. The Time 2 questionnaire was completed during their second semester at college. The questionnaire packet included standard questions regarding parents' and friends' influence on decisions about drinking,[31] and Zuckerman's sensation-seeking scale.[41] It also included the following description of a prototype and related instructions:

> The questions below concern "images"—that is, ideas that people have about typical members of different groups. For example, we all have ideas about what typical movie stars are like or what the typical grandmother is like. When asked, we might say that the typical movie star is pretty or rich, or that the typical grandmother is sweet and frail. We are not saying that all movie stars or all grandmothers are exactly alike, but rather that many

of them share certain characteristics. We would like you to think for a minute about the type of person (your age) who drinks alcohol frequently. How much do you think each of the following adjectives describes *your* image of that person?

These instructions were followed by 12 adjectives intended to assess the favorability of the image (e.g., smart, popular, careless, "cool," and self-centered). An additional question asked participants how similar they thought they were to the prototype. The mean of the 12 adjective favorability ratings was later multiplied by the similarity response to create a prototype index, hereafter referred to as prototype perception.

The primary criterion variable was a single item measure of alcohol frequency.*

How many times in the last 3 months have you had a whole drink of alcohol (for example, a bottle of beer, a glass of wine, or a whole mixed drink)?

A hierarchical regression analysis was employed to test the hypothesis that prototype perception would predict change in the frequency of alcohol use in this sample after social influences and sensation seeking had been entered into the equation. Thus, Time 1 alcohol use was entered into the equation first, followed by gender and sensation seeking. These were followed by the two social influence questions (friends' influence and parents' influence), and finally, the prototype perception. The criterion variable, of course, was alcohol use frequency at Time 2. The results of this regression analysis, which supported our hypotheses, are presented in Table 2. As can be seen in the table, Time 1 alcohol use and sensation seeking were significant predictors. Neither friends' influence

---

*Similar results have also been found with other drinking measures, such as the number of times the person has been drunk in the past 6 mo.

Table 2
Hierarchical Regression Results
Predicting Alcohol Use Among College Students[a]

Variable	β	t	p<
Time 1 alcohol use	.55	14.05	.001
Gender	−.01	<1	—
Sensation seeking	.09	2.84	.005
Friend influence	.05	1.64	—
Parent influence	−.03	−1.05	—
Prototype perception	.11	2.82	.005

[a]Final regression equation: $R^2 = .43$; $F(6, 611) = 78.19$, $p < .001$.

nor parents' influence made a significant contribution to predicting alcohol use among this sample. More important from the current perspective, students' perceptions of the prototypical drinker at Time 1 significantly predicted drinking at Time 2, even after the variance associated with Time 1 drinking, parent and peer influence, and sensation seeking had been removed.*

Adolescent Sample

Our second sample was included in an attempt to replicate these findings with a younger, less experienced group. Half of these adolescents were in the 8th grade and the other half were in the 10th grade at Time 1; they were in the 9th or 11th grade at Time 2. The same general categories of variables were used again, with one minor change in the measures. In addition to the influence question used with the college sample, two reaction questions were also asked: How

*Additional variables were also entered into the hierarchical regression, including: self-esteem, negative life events, parental drinking behaviors, and family financial problems. None of these made independent contributions to the regression equation.

Table 3
Hierarchical Regression Results
Predicting Alcohol Use Among Rural Adolescents[a]

Variable	β	t	p<
Time 1 alcohol use	.43	9.46	.001
Gender[b]	.06	1.77	.08
Sensation seeking	.11	3.10	.002
Friend Influence × Reaction	.13	3.27	.001
Parent Influence × Reaction	.04	.98	—
Prototype perception	.20	4.47	.001

[a]Final regression equation: $R^2 = .48$; $F(6, 444) = 69.61$, $p < .001$.
[b]Males were coded as a 1 and females were coded as a 2.

favorably or unfavorably would your friends and parents react if they knew you drank alcohol? The reaction scores were then multiplied by the influence score to create two influence indexes.

Once again, a hierarchical regression analysis was conducted regressing Time 2 alcohol use on the same variables. As in the previous study, Time 1 alcohol use was entered into the equation first, followed by gender and sensation seeking. This was followed by the Friends' (Reaction × Influence) Index, the Parents' (Reaction × Influence) Index, and the prototype perception. The criterion variable, once again, was frequency of alcohol use at Time 2. The results of this regression are presented in Table 3.

Consistent with the regression results from the college sample, Time 1 alcohol use, sensation seeking, and the alcohol prototype were significant predictors. In addition, the new influence of friends index did reach significance in this sample. More notable, however, is the fact that both studies supported our primary hypothesis: Perception of the prototypical drinker significantly predicts alcohol use, even when entered after all of the other predictor variables.

The Prototype

It is worth noting that, even though the alcohol proto-types of both the adolescents and the college students were strong predictors of their drinking behavior, in an absolute sense, these prototypes were not very favorable at all. In fact, both similarity and favorability ratings were consistently below the midpoint of the scale and they were much more negative than the ratings subjects gave to themselves on the same measures. This was true even among those who were currently drinking (although to a lesser extent, of course). What this suggests is that these students were not really trying to acquire a particular image. Instead, prototype favorability appears to be an indication of the adolescents' willingness to do a particular behavior, and, by so doing, be included in a distinctive and easily identifiable group (e.g., smoker or drinker).[54] In fact, results from our assessment of early or precocious sexual behavior and smoking suggests that very few adolescents intend to engage in a given risk behavior (or actually aspire to their associated images); rather, the prototype is an indication of their willingness to engage, should the opportunity present itself, in a particular behavior. This observation has implications for alcohol interventions, which we discuss later.

Alcohol Use and Sexual Behavior

Additional analyses from this project are relevant to the topic of this volume and therefore worth discussing here. One of the most overlooked, yet impactful, consequences of adolescent drinking is unprotected or casual sex. In order to assess the relation between alcohol use and sexual behaviors, we compared the sexual activity of drinkers and nondrinkers for the 6 mo preceding Time 1. For these analyses, we categorized both college students and adolescent participants as "nondrinkers" (those reporting drinking "never" or "once or twice") or "drinkers" (those reporting drinking "a few times"

Table 4
Alcohol Use and Sexual Behavior[a]

	Adolescent sample[b]		College sample[c]	
	Drinkers	Nondrinkers	Drinkers	Nondrinkers
Sexual intercourse				
Yes	33%	9%	73%	41%
No	67%	91%	27%	59%
n	74	424	401	278
	Sexually active adolescent sample[d]		Sexually active college sample[e]	
	Drinkers	Nondrinkers	Drinkers	Nondrinkers
Number of partners				
One partner	42%	57%	35%	64%
More than one	58%	43%	65%	36%
n	24	38	291	112

[a]These analyses were conducted on the Time 1 data. Reported chi-squares are likelihood ratios.

[b]$\chi^2(1, N = 498) = 25.9$, $p < .001$. [c]$\chi^2(1, N = 679) = 69.1$, $p < .001$. [d]$\chi^2(1, N = 62) = 1.01$, NS. [e]$\chi^2(1, N = 403) = 29.3$, $p < .001$.

or "regularly"). As can be seen in Table 4, there is a clear association between drinking and engaging in sexual intercourse in both groups. More specifically, the drinkers in both groups were significantly more likely than the nondrinkers to have engaged in sexual intercourse. In addition, the sexually active drinkers among the college students reported having significantly more sexual partners than did the nondrinking sexually active college students. (The pattern for the adolescents was the same, but the difference between drinking and nondrinking adolescents was not statistically significant, mostly because so few adolescents in our sample were sexually active.)

Several additional questions were asked of the college students to further investigate the association between drinking and sex. Responses to these questions also provide evidence of a correlation between alcohol use and risky sex. For example, 17% of the students indicated that drinking before sex had contributed to their failure to use birth control at least once in the last 6 mo. Twenty percent reported that drinking had contributed to their failure to use condoms some time during the last 6 mo. Perhaps most striking, however, is the fact that a full 25% reported that they had had too much to drink and then had sex with someone they had not intended to have sex with during the last 6 mo.

Conclusions

The current findings from our own research support three major conclusions. First, adolescent drinking is prevalent in rural areas just as it is in urban areas. Second, teenagers in rural areas, like those in urban areas, are more likely to drink if they have a general inclination toward sensation seeking than if they do not. And third, adolescents' social cognitions, specifically their perceptions of the prototypical drinker, are a significant factor in their decisions to drink. Because the first two of these conclusions are not entirely novel, and the prototype perceptions do represent a new approach to understanding adolescent drinking, we focus our discussion here on the applications of this finding for research and intervention.

Applications of the Prototype Perception Approach

One obvious question regarding the prototype is whether changes in these perceptions are related to changes in adolescent drinking. Our data suggest that such an assumption is justified. More specifically, additional analyses of the longitudinal data from both our college and adolescent samples have indicated that perceptions of the prototype "track" changes in drinking behavior quite closely.[55] Among freshmen, students who reported more positive perceptions of the proto-typical drinker in their second semester than they had in their first semester also reported an increase in the amount of drinking done during that same period. Furthermore, those whose perceptions of the prototype became more negative reported decreased drinking over this period of time. These results are consistent with our findings from research with smokers,[58] and this effect has been replicated with the adolescent sample. In short, the link between adolescents' perceptions of the drinker prototype and their drinking behavior appears to be a strong one. Moreover, that link is both prospective and reactive—perceptions signal a change in drinking behavior but they also react to, or change as a result of, increases or decreases in drinking behavior.

Prototype Modification

What this suggests is that efforts to alter the favorability and structure of the prototype may very well prove effective at deterring, or at least delaying, onset of adolescent alcohol use. More specifically, efforts to both distance from and dero-gate the prototypical drinker, perhaps by associating early alcohol use with unappealing or distasteful characterizations, may prove effective. In this regard, the fact that the alcohol prototype is not very favorable in an absolute sense is encour-aging. In particular, certain characteristics attributed to the prototype are not flattering at all (e.g., not very smart, imma-ture, and inconsiderate). It would appear that educators could take advantage of these perceptions by amplifying—or actu-ally exacerbating—these negative characteristics. In so doing, it may be possible to significantly reduce the number of ado-lescents who find the image acceptable, and therefore are will-ing to go along when others start drinking, smoking, or engaging in other risk behaviors. Given the importance of images in determining behavior, this approach strikes us as one that is easily implemented, relatively speaking, and more important, potentially quite fruitful.

Methodological Advantages

In addition to these potential applications of prototype perception to interventions, the development of the construct has a variety of methodological advantages. Foremost among these is the fact that the prototype is an indirect measure of favorability toward risky behavior, and therefore is less vulnerable to social desirability and response bias than are more direct measures.[56] An adolescent may be very reluctant to admit to positive attitudes toward drinking—or may even be unaware of such attitudes, but still reveal positive opinions, or at least an acceptance of the drinker prototype, which suggests preintentional inclinations. Another advantage is that the format of the prototype perception questions (i.e., rating adjectives as descriptive of the prototype) lends itself to comparison between the participant's self-perceptions and prototype perception, or ideal-self perceptions and prototype perceptions. Such comparisons can be valuable in determining how self-perceptions (vis-à-vis the prototype) factor into the decision to drink.

A number of questions about the prototype remain. Perhaps foremost among these is the question of how difficult it is to modify prototypes. We are not aware of any experimental efforts to modify images or prototypes (although a number of antismoking and antidrug campaigns have taken this approach). Given changes in public perception of smoking and smokers over the last decade, however, there is reason for optimism. A related, and equally important question, because of its implications for intervention, has to do with how and when these prototypes develop. In this regard, it has been shown that even grade school children have clear and distinct images of smokers;[59,60] in most cases these images come from exposure to portrayals of smokers in print, on television, and in films.[53] We also suspect that parents and peers are important sources of prototypes, and believe that it is important to investigate their role in the initial formation of prototypes, as well as their role in altering prototypes to decrease adolescent drinking.

Summary and Implications

The next step after identifying where and how adolescents develop their prototypes is then to attack both the favorability and acceptability of these images. That is, denigrate the typical drinker prototype, making it less favorable and, therefore, unacceptable. This could be done by presenting actual data, such as the fact that typical drinkers are also much more likely to drop out of school, participate in fewer extracurricular activities, have worse family relations, and engage in other risk behaviors.[13] Perhaps just in the mere discussion of images, the favorability and acceptance may diminish. The idea of prototypes in preventive programs could also be generalized to other risk behaviors. For example, the image of the reckless and/or drunk driver is another prototype that could be attacked in an educational setting and made less favorable. This, once again, could be accomplished by showing the risks associated with the behaviors. Whereas the favorability of the typical drinker and reckless, drunk driver needs to be reduced, enhancing the favorability and acceptance of other prototypes would be beneficial. For example, increasing the favorability and acceptance of the typical condom user would actually increase the chances that adolescents would use condoms. If the typical condom user was seen as intelligent, popular, and "cool"; and if using condoms was thought to be the norm, more adolescents would likely engage in this protective behavior.

References

[1]T. L. Napier, T. J. Carter, and M. C. Pratt (1981) Correlates of alcohol and marijuana use among rural high school students. *Rural Sociol.* **46,** 319–332.

[2]Iowa Department of Public Health (1988) *Vital Statistics of Iowa.* Author, Des Moines, IA.

[3]R. Blum (1987) Contemporary threats to adolescent health in the United Sates. *JAMA* **257,** 3390–3395.

[4]National Center for Health Statistics (1987) *Vital Statistics of the US, 1987, Vol. I. Natality.* DHHS Pub. No. (PHS) 89-1100, Public Health Service, US Government Printing Office, Washington, DC.

[5]G. M. Barnes (1977) The development of adolescent drinking behavior: an evaluative review of the impact of the socialization process within the family. *Adolescence* **12,** 572–589.

[6]E. H. Erikson (1950) *Childhood and Society.* Norton, New York.

[7]E. R. Oetting and F. Beauvais (1990) Adolescent drug use: findings of national and local surveys. *J. Consult. Clin. Psychol.* **58,** 385–394.

[8]R. H. Coombs and M. J. Paulson (1988) Contrasting family patterns of adolescent drug users and nonusers. *J. Chem. Depend. Treatment* **1,** 59–72.

[9]S. Keys and J. Block (1984) Prevalence and patterns of substance use among early adolescents. *J. Youth Adolescence* **13,** 1–14.

[10]P. M. Kingery, E. Mirzaee, B. E. Pruitt, R. S. Hurley, and G. Heuberger (1991) Rural communities near large metropolitan areas: safe havens from adolescent violence and drug use? *Health Values: J. Health Behav. Educ. Promotion* **15,** 39–48.

[11]P. D. Sarvella and E. J. McClendon (1987) Early adolescent alcohol abuse in rural northern Michigan. *Community Mental Health J.* **23,** 183–191.

[12]R. Swaim, F. Beauvais, R. W. Edwards, and E. R. Oetting (1986) Adolescent drug use in three small rural communities in the Rocky Mountain region. *J. Drug Educ.* **16,** 57–73.

[13]L. P. Bloch, L. S. Crockett, and J. R. Vicary (1991) Antecedents of rural adolescent alcohol use: a risk factor approach. *J. Drug Educ.* **21,** 361–377.

[14]R. Jessor and R. Jessor (1977) *Problem Behavior: A Longitudinal Study of Youth.* Academic, New York.

[15]D. M. Donovan and A. G. Marlatt (1982) Personality subtypes among driving while intoxicated offenders: relationship to drinking behavior and driving risk. *J. Consult. Clin. Psychol.* **50,** 241–249.

[16]B. F. Banahan and D. J. McCaffrey (1993) Rural students' exposure to risk from automobile travel when the driver is under the influence of alcohol or drugs. *J. Rural Health* **9,** 50–56.

[17]J. E. Donovan and R. Jessor (1985) Structure of problem behavior in adolescence and young adulthood. *J. Consult. Clin. Psychol.* **53,** 890–904.

[18]L. Strunin and R. Hingson (1992) Alcohol, drugs, and adolescent sexual behavior. *Int. J. Addict.* **27,** 129–146.

[19]B. Flanigan, A. McLean, C. Hall, and V. Propp (1990) Alcohol use as a situational influence on young women's pregnancy risk-taking behaviors. *Adolescence* **25,** 205–214.

[20]T. C. Harford and G. S. Mills (1978) Age-related trends in alcohol consumption. *J. Student Alcohol.* **39,** 207–210.

[21]J. W. Graham, G. Marks, and W. B. Hansen (1991) Social influence processes affecting adolescent substance use. *J. Appl. Psychol.* **76,** 291–298.

[22]R. Z. Margulies, R. C. Kessler, and D. B. Kandel (1977) A longitudinal study of onset of drinking among high school students. *Q. J. Stud. Alcohol* **38,** 879–912.

[23]R. G. Smart and G. Gray (1979) Parental and peer influences as correlates of problem drinking among high school students. *Int. J. Addict.* **14,** 905–918.

[24]R. G. Smart, G. Gray, and C. Bennett (1978) Predictors of drinking and signs of heavy drinking among high school students. *Int. J. Addict.* **13,** 1079–1094.

[25]B. J. Biddle, B. J. Bank, and M. M. Marlin (1980) Social determinants of adolescent drinking: what they think, what they do and what I think and do. *J. Stud. Alcohol* **41,** 215–241.

[26]T. Hirschi (1969) *Causes of Delinquency.* University of California Press, Berkeley, CA.

[27]R. D. Hays, A. W. Stacy, K. F. Widaman, M. R. DiMatteo, and R. Downey (1986) Multistage path models of adolescent alcohol and drug use: a reanalysis. *J. Drug Issues* **16,** 357–369.

[28]S. Gibbons, M. L. Wylie, L. Echterling, and J. French (1986) Situational factors related to rural adolescent alcohol use. *Int. J. Addict.* **21,** 1183–1195.

[29]J. E. Pendorf (1992) Leisure time use and academic correlates of alcohol abuse among high school students. *J. Alcohol Drug Educ.* **37,** 103–110.

[30]I. Ajzen and M. Fishbein (1980) *Understanding Attitudes and Predicting Social Behavior.* Prentice-Hall, Englewood Cliffs, NJ.

[31]M. Fishbein and I. Ajzen (1975) *Belief, Attitude, Intention, and Behavior: An Introduction to Theory and Research.* Addison-Wesley, Reading, MA.

[32]B. B. Brown, D. R. Classen, and S. A. Eicher (1986) Perceptions of peer pressure, peer conformity dispositions, and self-reported behavior among adolescents. *Dev. Psychol.* **22,** 521–530.

[33]D. S. Elliott, S. S. Ageton, D. Huizingo, B. A. Knowles, and R. J. Canter (1983) *The Prevalence and Incidence of Delinquent Behavior: 1976–1980.* Behavioral Research Institute, Boulder, CO.

[34]T. E. Dielman, P. C. Campanelli, J. T. Shope, and A. T. Butchart (1987) Susceptibility to peer pressure, self-esteem, and health locus of control as correlates of adolescent substance abuse. *Health Educ. Q.* **14,** 207–221.

[35]F. X. Gibbons, M. Helweg-Larsen, and M. Gerrard (in press) Prevalence estimates and adolescent risk behavior: cross cultural differences in social influence. *J. Applied Psychol.*

[36]R. D. Conger, F. O. Lorenz, G. H. Elder, J. N. Melby, R. L. Simmons, and K. J. Conger (1991) A process model of family economic pressure and early adolescent alcohol use. *J. Early Adolescence* **11,** 430–449.

[37]R. R. Kafka and P. London (1991) Communication in relationships and adolescent substance use: the influence of parents and friends. *Adolescence* **26,** 587–598.

[38]G. H. Elder (1974) *Children of the Great Depression: Social Change in Life Experience.* University of Chicago Press, Chicago.

[39]A. Eskilson, M. G. Wiley, G. Muehlbauer, and L. Dodder (1986) Parental pressure, self-esteem, and adolescent reported deviance: bending the twig too far. *Adolescence* **21,** 501–515.

[40]J. E. Donovan and R. Jessor (1983) Problem drinking in adolescence and young adulthood: a follow-up study. *J. Stud. Alcohol* **44,** 109–137.

[41]M. Zuckerman (1979) *Sensation Seeking: Beyond the Optimal Level of Arousal.* Erlbaum, Hillsdale, NJ.

[42]M. D. Newcomb and P. M. Bentler (1986) Frequency and sequence of drug use: a longitudinal study from early adolescence to young adulthood. *J. Drug Educ.* **16,** 101–120.

[43]A. W. Stacy, M. C. Newcomb, and P. M. Bentler (1993) Cognitive motivations and sensation-seeking as long-term predictors of drinking problems. *J. Soc. Clin. Psychol.* **12,** 1–24.

[44]K. Baker, J. Beer, and J. Beer (1991) Self-esteem, alcoholism, sensation seeking, GPA, and differential aptitude test scores of high school students in an honor society. *Psychol. Rep.* **69,** 1147–1150.

[45]G. A. Marlatt and D. J. Rohsenow (1980) Cognitive processes in alcohol use: expectancy and the balanced-placebo design, in *Advances in Substance Abuse: Behavioral and Biological Research, Vol. 1.* N. K. Mello, ed. JAI Press, Greenwich, CT, pp. 159–199.

[46]G. J. Connors and S. A. Maisto (1988) The alcohol expectancy construct: overview and clinical applications. *Cogn. Ther. Res.* **12,** 487–504.

[47]L. McLaughlin-Mann, L. Chassin, and K. J. Sher (1987) Alcohol expectancies and the risk for alcoholism. *J. Consult. Clin. Psychol.* **55,** 411–417.

[48]M. S. Goldman, S. A. Brown, and B. A. Christiansen (1987) Expectancy theory: thinking about drinking, in *Psychological Theories of Drinking and Alcoholism.* H. T. Blane and K. E. Leonard, eds. Guilford, New York, pp. 181–226.

[49]B. C. Leigh (1989) In search of the seven dwarves: issues of measurement and meaning in alcohol expectancy research. *Psychol. Bull.* **105,** 361–373.

[50]L. Chassin, C. C. Presson, S. J. Sherman, E. Corty, and R. W. Olshavsky (1981) Self-images and cigarette smoking in adolescence. *Pers. Soc. Psychol. Bull.* **7,** 670–676.

[51]L. Chassin, C. C. Presson, and S. J. Sherman (1990) Social psychological contributions to the understanding and prevention of adolescent cigarette smoking. *Pers. Soc. Psychol. Bull.* **16,** 133–151.

[52]L. Chassin, C. Tetzloff, and M. Hershey (1985) Self-image and social-image factors in adolescent alcohol use. *J. Stud. Alcohol* **46,** 39–47.

[53]H. Leventhal and P. D. Cleary (1980) The smoking problem: a review of the research and theory in behavioral risk modification. *Psychol. Bull.* **88,** 370–405.

[54]F. X. Gibbons and M. Gerrard (in press) Social comparison and social behaviors: a prototype model of risk behavior, in *Health, Cop-*

ing, and Social Comparison. B. Buunk and F. X. Gibbons, eds. Erlbaum, Hillsdale, NJ.

[55]F. X. Gibbons and M. Gerrard (in press) Predicting young adult's health risk behavior. *J. Pers. Soc. Psychol.*

[56]F. X. Gibbons, M. Gerrard, and S. Boney-McCoy (in press) Prototype perception predicts (lack of) pregnancy prevention. *Pers. Soc. Psychol. Bull.*

[57]F. X. Gibbons, C. P. Benbow, and M. Gerrard (1994) From top dog to bottom half: strategies in response to poor performance. *J. Pers. Soc. Psychol.* **67**, 638–652.

[58]F. X. Gibbons, M. Gerrard, H. A. Lando, and P. G. McGovern (1991) Social comparison and smoking cessation: the role of the "typical smoker." *J. Exp. Soc. Psychol.* **27**, 239–258.

[59]M. J. Bland, B. R. Bewley, and I. Day (1975) Primary schoolboys: image of self and smoker. *Br. J. Prev. Soc. Med.* **29**, 262–266.

[60]J. M. Bynner (1970) Behavioral research into children's smoking: some implications for anti-smoking strategy. *R. Soc. Health J.* **90**, 159–163.

The Role of Culture in Preventing Perinatal Abuse of Alcohol and Other Drugs

Vivian L. Smith

Introduction

Experience from projects sponsored by the United States Center for Substance Abuse Prevention (CSAP) indicates that culture can play a critical role in developing programs that prevent the perinatal abuse of alcohol and other drugs (AOD), including tobacco. The first priority in prevention and treatment is reaching the targeted population—getting their attention and gaining their trust. This first priority seems obvious enough, but in the current debate over cultural competence, the obvious is easily obscured by both the magnitude of the problem and the fear of losing professional status. Well-intentioned programs abound that complain the familiar refrain, "We tried to help them but they didn't want the help

From: *Drug and Alcohol Abuse Reviews, Vol. 8:*
Drug and Alcohol Abuse During Pregnancy and Childhood
Ed.: R. R. Watson ©1995 Humana Press Inc., Totowa, NJ

or they wouldn't come." Early lessons learned from CSAP-funded projects indicate that some gaps in program design and effectiveness can be bridged by cultural competence. CSAP's working definition of cultural competence is:

> a set of academic and interpersonal skills that allow individuals to increase their understanding and appreciation of cultural differences and similarities within, among and between groups. This requires a willingness and ability to draw upon community based values, traditions and customs to work with knowledgeable persons and from the community in developing focused interventions, communications and other support.[1]

Cultural competence can be a sensitive issue with health care professionals. Many professionals in the prevention and treatment communities fear cultural competence as a racial litmus test, i.e., if you are not African American, Asian, Latino, or Native American you cannot develop programs that help African Americans, Asians, Latinos, or Native Americans. Cultural competence is a far richer concept defined not by exclusion, but by inclusion. It is critical that fear of losing professional status does not dominate the debate and obscure the potential benefits of programs addressing the cultural needs of targeted populations where the abuse of alcohol, tobacco, and other drugs continue to threaten the health of generations.

CSAP Background

CSAP's major funding initiative for pregnant women and their babies is the Pregnant Postpartum Women and Their Infants Demonstration Grant (PPWI). PPWI started in 1989 and has since funded 148 grants for a total of $135,469,000. The mostly 5 yr grants have served approx 8766 women and 3289 infants, focusing largely on primary and secondary prevention with services ranging from prevention to treatment. In its legislative mandate, PPWI was charged with the responsibility of assuring development of innovative programs for low-income women and their infants. Most of the programs were developed in community-based organizations, academic institutions, and other prevention and treatment organizations. They are in urban environments with a smaller number of rural and suburban PPWI grants. As these environments are different, so too must be the prevention strategies to reach the targeted populations. PPWI has recognized the often critical role of culture in program design and development. PPWI funding initiatives therefore have targeted African Americans, Asians, Hispanics, and Native Americans for innovative approaches to prevention and treatment.

The Case for Cultural Competence

Examining the scope of the AOD problems facing women in the ethnic/racial communities points to the need for culturally based interventions. Although AOD use among ethnic/racial populations is generally lower than Whites, extreme use among African Americans, Asians, and Native Americans is higher. So are the resulting infant mortality rates. Annually, some 375,000 infants are born to women who use alcohol and other drugs, including tobacco, during their pregnancies.[2,3] Many of these babies are born prematurely, and if carried to term, are often underweight. Fetal Alcohol Syndrome (FAS) is 33 times more likely among Native Americans than Whites. The rate of FAS and its accompanying mental retardation is 6.7 times higher for Black women than White women. Clearly, AOD abuse among pregnant women is a widespread problem. It is worse in some ethnic/racial communities where women often do not go to doctors. Two of the reasons suggested are poverty—they cannot afford to transport themselves to health care facilities—and the lack of culturally unacceptable services.[4] In a social learning analysis of the plight of many ethnic/racial pregnant women, both reasons for their not accessing health care can be viewed as a function of the environmental factors that dictate their lives. In order to help prevent AOD abuse, it is necessary to first understand, without judging and without imposing values.

The cycle of AOD use by pregnant women abusing their bodies and their unborn babies is often determined by cultural values and norms. Children born of mothers who used drugs during pregnancy are more likely to use drugs themselves. Obviously, they value AOD in a way different from women who do not use drugs. What is less obvious to many in the fields of prevention and treatment is that simply offering pregnant women a drug free life (often outside of their familiar environments), does not negate the values, norms, attitudes, and experiences that influence their pattern of drug use. These cultural issues must be taken into account for effective prevention and treatment. Prevention and treatment of drug addiction is far more complex than just getting addicts to say "no." Their particular problems often do not go away when they are drug free because their environments do not go away. Even without drugs, often pregnant women from some ethnic/racial communities will still be poor, unemployed, or discriminated against. They may still be without adequate housing, still live in violent environments, and still be daughters of addicted persons. Successful interventions must not only address the reasons why but also identify the cultural supports required to sustain the benefits of any intervention.

The reasons for AOD drug abuse among ethnic/racial populations may differ from the circumstances that drive Whites to drugs. For instance, during high school, Black teenagers drink less than White teenagers. After high school, drinking among Blacks rises, surpassing drinking rates among Whites. Also, after high school, poor Blacks come face to face with a bleak economic future. Study after study has documented exceptionally high rates of Black teenage unemployment. An obvious hypothesis is that the increased drinking rate among Blacks has some correlation to the hopelessness and despair attendant with unemployment. In other words, when faced with nothing to do after high school, many Blacks turn to the bottle. High unemployment and high rates of alcoholism also go hand in hand in many Native American communities.

Successful alcohol treatment has established that finding an alcoholic a job produces good long-term results. Applying this general finding to the specific circumstances of African American or Native American alcoholics requires not only a cultural analysis of the problem, but a reality check in solving it. Given that Black and Native American unemployment is significantly higher than that for Whites, what we know to be a successful intervention, namely a job, is sometimes an impractical solution in the increased alcoholism among Blacks and Native Americans. Again, a cultural analysis is required to develop a realistic intervention.

AOD issues among Asian and Hispanic populations often require a unique cultural analysis. For instance, immigration and language problems often need to be addressed. Bilingual staff is the most obvious need. Perhaps an even greater need in developing effective prevention and treatment strategies is recognizing that heterogeneity of Asian and Hispanic cultural norms in the US can vary significantly. For instance, the environmental pressures on an acculturated third generation Japanese American using drugs are not likely to be the same as those on a recent Filipino immigrant, any more than one can assume that a prevention strategy effectively targeting pregnant Puerto Rican women will effectively meet the AOD prevention needs of women who just recently fled war-torn El Salvador. The values, norms, and experiences of each group will shape their pattern of drug use and the strategies required for prevention and treatment.

Ethnic/racial women abusing AOD, including pregnant women, often complain that they do not feel comfortable when they go for treatment administered by Whites based on assumptions about Whites. The result is that they generally do not go to treatment and have not benefited from AOD strategies that ignore their cultural needs. Very often part of their problem is a need to talk about and develop strategies for coping with racism. Given the tendency of many White professionals to try to ignore racism in favor of more color blind humanistic approaches, a critical need of ethnic/racial populations is often overlooked in developing prevention and treatment strategies for AOD abuse.

The need to develop long-term strategies that address particular AOD needs in racial/ethnic communities require both an understanding of the weaknesses and strengths of those communities. Clinical approaches have limited success without environmental strategies. Time out from individual problems, be it counseling, training, or some other intervention, is limited to short-lived results when individuals are thrown back into environments that help create the problems. Yet, often these environments have untapped supports.

Several CSAP-funded projects build on cultural strengths rather than assume cultural deficits. The Granny House, for instance, operates in a housing project in Atlanta, GA. Grandmothers are trained and certified as foster parents of children with drug-abusing mothers. Instead of applying a cultural analysis defined by weakness, i.e., talking about broken homes and the absence of fathers, the project builds on a strength of the African-American experience. The program developers hypothesized that women who had lovingly raised their children and their grandchildren might have the experience and compassion to help the children of women abusing drugs. The Young Families Support Program in Boston, MA focuses on the practical problems, like housing and day care, that affect the drug habits of adolescent mothers. A CSAP PPWI program in Gainesville, FL, uses Resource Mothers to recruit drug-abusing women into the program. These paraprofessionals are from the targeted community and make regular home visits to pregnant women, encouraging them to get health care while helping them to resolve problems specific to their cultural needs. The Resource Mothers say they are careful not to judge, not to put down, and not to push the drug-abusing mothers into unwanted school programs. They say the result is that more of them choose to go to school, go to the doctor, and ask for other help. In all three of the projects mentioned, multicultural staff administer interdisciplinary programs where cultural sensitivity is a key element of success.

Despite the success of culturally sensitive interventions in preventing pregnant women from AOD abuse, controversy among professionals over cultural competence simmers. Much of the resistance is unstated—private conversations and determined unwillingness to further the research. The fears of professionals is in some ways comparable to the culturally based fears of ethnic/racial groups, where pregnant women are reluctant to go to the doctor. Both view change as threatening a way of life that they do not recognize the need to challenge. For many AOD professionals at universities and in the field, administering projects to the needy is their livelihood. They are the experts. They view cultural competence as threatening both their livelihood and their status. It is understandable but not acceptable.

Summary

AOD abuse of pregnant women in racial and ethnic communities is a problem too costly to society to ignore. Researchers and professionals cannot afford to ignore approaches that show promise. Whether called cultural sensitivity, cultural competence, or just plain respect for other people's culture, it is time to further the research, particularly as we become more and more a multicultural society. Cultural competence should not frighten professionals in the field of AOD prevention and treatment. It is an opportunity to expand our understanding rather than limit our thinking to approaches that do not reach, let alone help, the population often in greatest need.

CSAP has taken a lead in funding programs that incorporate cultural sensitivity into program design and administration. Some will demonstrate more success than others. Cultural competence is not a substitute for commitment and sound project design, but it is a needy addition.

References

[1]M. A. Orlandi, R. Westson, and L. G. Epstein (eds.) (1992) *Cultural Competence for Evaluators: A Guide for Alcohol and Other Drug Abuse Prevention Practitioners Working with Ethnic/Racial Communities.* Public Health Service, Alcohol, Drug Abuse, and Mental Health Administration, Office for Substance Abuse Prevention, US Department of Health and Human Services (USDHHS # ADM-92-1884), Rockville, MD.

[2]Center for Substance Abuse Prevention (1993) *Pregnancy and Exposure to Alcohol and Other Drug Use.* Division of Demonstrations for High Risk Populations, US Department of Health and Human Services, Rockville, MD.

[3]Center for Substance Abuse Prevention (1993) *Toward Preventing Perinatal Abuse of Alcohol and Other Drugs.* Division of Demonstrations for High Risk Populations, US Department of Health and Human Services, Rockville, MD.

[4]J. P. Butler (1992) Of kindred minds: the ties that bind, in *Cultural Competence for Evaluators: A Guide for Alcohol and Other Drug Abuse Prevention Practitioners Working with Ethnic/Racial Communities.* M. A. Orlandi, R. Westson, and L. G. Epstein, eds. Public Health Service, Alcohol, Drug Abuse, and Mental Health Administration, Office for Substance Abuse Prevention, US Department of Health and Human Services (USDHHS # ADM-92-1884), Rockville, MD.

Bibliography

M. Aguirre-Molina (1991) Issues for Latinos: Puerto Rican women, in *Alcohol and Drugs Are Women's Issues, Volume 1—A Review of the Issues.* P. Roth, ed. Women's Action Alliance and the Scarecrow Press, Inc., Metuchen, NJ, pp. 93–100.

D. R. Arkinson, G. Morton, and D. W. Sue (1979) *Minority Identity Development. Counseling and American Minorities: A Cross-Cultural Perspective, 1–4.* Brown, Dubuque, IA.

Avance, Inc. (1986) *Minority Families Preventing Child Abuse and Neglect Through Parenting Education.* Author, San Antonio, TX.

J. G. Bachman, J. M. Wallace, P. M. O'Malley, L. D. Johnston, C. L. Kurth, and H. W. Neighbors (1991) Racial/ethnic differences in smoking, drinking, and illicit drug use among American high school seniors, 1976–89. *Am. J. Public Health* **81(3),** 372–377.

R. Beauvais and J. E. Trimble (1992) *The Role of the Researcher in Evaluating American Indian Alcohol and Other Drug Preventing Programs.* Cultural Competence for Evaluators, 173-201, DHHS No. ADM-92-1884, National Clearinghouse for Alcohol and Drug Information, Rockville, MD.

A. B. Berenson, N. H. Stiglich, G. S. Wilkinson, and G. D. Anderson (1991) Drug abuse and other risk factors for physical abuse in pregnancy among White Non-Hispanic, Black, and Hispanic women. *Am. J. Obstet. Gynecol.* **164(6),** 1491–1499.

M. S. Boone (1985) Social and cultural factors in the etiology of low birth weight among disadvantaged blacks. *Soc. Sci. Med.* **20(10),** 1001–1011.

J. M. Casas (1992) *A Culturally Sensitive Model for Evaluating Alcohol and Other Drug Abuse Prevention Programs: A Hispanic Perspective.* Cultural Competence for Evaluators (DHHS No. ADM-92-1884), National Clearinghouse for Alcohol and Drug Information, Rockville, MD.

C. G. Coll (1992) *Cultural Diversity: Implications for Theory and Practice.* Manuscript submitted for publication.

T. Cross (1991) *Working Toward Cultural Competence: One Agency's Experience.* American Professional Society on the Abuse of Children, Chicago.

T. I. Cross and I. Hansel (1986) *Positive Indian Parenting: Honoring Our Children by Honoring Our Traditions.* The Northwest Indian Child Welfare Institute., The Parry Center for Children, Portland, OR.

R. H. Dana (1988) *Assessment and Intervention Services for Multicultural Populations.* University of Arkansas, Little Rock.

R. L. Davis, S. D. Halgerson, and P. Waller (1992) Smoking during pregnancy among northwest Native Americans. *Public Health Rep.* **67,** 66–69.

M. M. Dore and A. O. Dumois (1990) Cultural differences in the meaning of adolescent pregnancy. *J. Contemp. Hum. Serv.* **71,** 93–101.

J. Gates-Williams, M. N. Jackson, V. Jenkins-Monroe, and L. R. Williams (1982) The business of preventing African-American infant mortality. *J. West. Med.* **157(3),** 350–356.

M. H. Gilbert (1991) Acculturation and changes in drinking patterns among Mexican-American women: implications for prevention. *Alcohol Health Res. World* **15(3),** 234–238.

C. J. Hogue and M. A. Hargraves (1993) *Class, Race, and Infant.* Emory University School of Public Health, Atlanta, GA.

R. A. LaDue (1991) Coyote returns: survival for Native American women, in *Alcohol and Drugs Are Women's Issues, Volume 1—A Review of the Issues.* P. Roth, ed. Women's Action Alliance and the Scarecrow Press, Inc., Metuchen, NJ, pp. 23–30.

T. J. Mann (1990) *Drawing on Cultural Strengths to Empower Families. Protecting Children, 3–5.* Child Welfare League of America, Washington, DC.

J. Mora and M. H. Gilbert (1991) Issues for Latinos: Mexican American women, in *Alcohol and Drugs Are Women's Issues, Volume 1—A Review of the Issues.* P. Roth, ed. Women's Action Alliance and the Scarecrow Press, Inc., Metuchen, NJ, pp. 43–47.

R. M. Nakamura, R. King, E. H. Kimball, R. K. Oye, and S. D. Helgerson (1990) Excess infant mortality in an American Indian population. *JAMA* **266(16),** 2244–2248.

People of Color Leadership Institute (1993) *Training Guidebook for Developing Cultural Competence.* Author, Washington, DC.

P. A. Poma (1987) Pregnancy in Hispanic women. *JAMA* **79(9),** 929–935.

L. Ramer (1992) Culturally sensitive caregiving and childbearing families, in *Nursing Issues for the 21st Century.* B. S. Raff and E. Fiore, eds. March of Dimes Foundation, White Plains, NY.

E. Randall-David (1989) *Strategies for Working with Culturally Diverse Communities and Clients.* Comprehensive Hemophilia Program, Bowman Gray School of Medicine, Association for the Care of Children's Health, Washington, DC.

L. Remez (1992) Infant mortality on an Oregon Indian reservation is almost three times higher than the overall U.S. rate. *Fam. Plan. Prospect.* **24(3),** 138,139.

L. S. Snyder (1992) *Fetal Alcohol Syndrome Resource Guide.* Indian Health Service, Albuquerque, NM.

C. J. Stephens (1987) The effects of social support on alcohol consumption during pregnancy: situational and ethnic/cultural considerations. *Int. J. Addict.* **22(7),** 609–619.

A. Sun (1991) Issues for Asian American women, in *Alcohol and Drugs Are Women's Issues, Volume 1—A Review of the Issues.* P. Roth, ed. Women's Action Alliance and the Scarecrow Press, Inc., Metuchen, NJ, pp. 125–128.

A. H. Taha-Cisse (1991) Issues for African American women, in *Alcohol and Drugs Are Women's Issues, Volume 1—A Review of the Issues.* P. Roth, ed. Women's Action Alliance and the Scarecrow Press, Inc., Metuchen, NJ, pp. 54–60.

C. W. Turner (1987) *Clinical Applications of the Store Center Theoretical Approach to Minority Women.* Manuscript submitted for publication.

S. Yen (1992) *Cultural Competence for Evaluators Working with Asian/Pacific Island-American Communities.* Cultural Competence for Evaluators (DHHS No. ADM-92-1884), National Clearinghouse for Alcohol and Drug Information, Rockville, MD.

Trends and Theories Concerning Alcohol and Other Drug Use Among Adolescent Females

*R. J. Russac
and Sharon T. Weaver*

Give me a girl at an impressionable age, and she is mine for life.

Muriel Spark

Introduction

Although attention in recent years has focused on optimistic reports of declining adolescent drug use,[1,2] some evidence suggests that alcohol and other substance use may actually be increasing among select subgroups. One group of particular concern is adolescent females. The reasons for placing adolescent females among those "at-risk" are varied and complex. However, it can be said that, along with measured

From: *Drug and Alcohol Abuse Reviews, Vol. 8:*
Drug and Alcohol Abuse During Pregnancy and Childhood
Ed.: R. R. Watson ©1995 Humana Press Inc., Totowa, NJ

progress toward equal opportunities for both sexes, there have appeared a new set of problems associated with changing roles, opportunities, and expectations for females.

We examine drug use behavior among adolescent females from three perspectives in this chapter. First, we focus on the assessment of substance use among adolescents in general, and adolescent females in particular. Second, we review findings from surveys of adolescent drug use, drawing heavily on our own efforts in this regard. Third, we examine the issue of causality with regard to drug use among adolescent females— first in terms of individual risk factors and then from four broad theoretical perspectives that attempt to integrate the correlates of substance use. Our goal in this chapter is not to provide a complete picture of a complex and rapidly evolving field, but rather to characterize the *zeitgeist* that is currently guiding our prevention, treatment, and research efforts. We also attempt to point out gaps in our knowledge base and areas of disagreement among professionals that must be addressed; doing so will lead us closer to an understanding of substance abuse among the young and how it can be prevented.

Problems of Assessment

The assessment of drug use raises a number important methodological issues. Some of these concerns are applicable to all populations, others are unique to adolescents, and still others specific to adolescent females. In this section, several assessment issues germane to adolescent drug use are reviewed. However, the problem of appropriate methodology is both subtle and perplexing, requiring a discussion well beyond the scope of this chapter.

Populations Assessed

Beginning in the early 1970s, drug use studies moved away from examining small, extreme populations (e.g., hard-core heroin addicts and chronic alcoholics) and toward an emphasis on substance use among larger, more representative samples of the population. Today most ongoing data collection efforts are presented in a manner that actually excludes special populations. For example, the *National Household Survey,* based on biannual interviews of individuals 12 yr and older from intact families, omits transients who might be expected to engage more frequently in substance use. Likewise, the *Michigan Study,* which has monitored drug use among high school seniors and young adults since 1971 (and more recently has expanded to include students in the 8th and 10th grades) fails to provide data on school dropouts and students with high absenteeism. Today most substance use data are collected on adolescent populations using instruments administered in traditional educational settings and therefore represent mainstream students in the middle-class school system, viz., those most amenable to and available for testing.

The effects of this sampling bias are unclear. Some prevention specialists suggest that recently reported declines in drug use among adolescents, if indeed they exist, are being observed only among adolescents least likely to engage in serious drug use. They question whether declining drug use rates among these adolescents can realistically be generalized to important "at-risk" populations that are conspicuous by their absence from most school-based surveys. Other researchers argue cogently that the recent emphasis on use patterns among normal populations has produced several benefits. Kandel[3] suggested that, because severely addicted individuals represent only a small proportion of the population (particularly among youth), their exclusion from the database does not significantly affect "absolute epidemiological estimates reported" (p. 240). Moreover, a focus on representative samples of student populations, she believes, has led to a more realistic picture of the overall drug problem among young people. As an

example, Kandel pointed out that studies of extreme populations (e.g., individuals who have been incarcerated or identified in clinical settings) present a picture of addiction that is
progressive and irreversible. However, studies of "mainstream" adolescents provide a more optimistic view, one that
has "led to fundamental revisions in our understanding of
extreme forms of drug involvement such as alcoholism or
heroin addiction" (p. 240). One fact not in debate is that data
from special populations have yet to be adequately integrated
with data gathered from mainstream student populations.

Method of Reporting

Another characteristic of current adolescent drug surveys
is that they rely almost entirely on students' self-reports of
drug use. We would be very trusting indeed simply to assume
that such reports are accurate.[4] Inaccuracies in self-reported
data are derived from two primary sources: Students who
underemphasize their drug use and students who overemphasize their drug use. Some students, particularly those who
believe that discovery of their use of an illicit substance will
lead to strong disciplinary or legal consequences, are likely to
understate their involvement with drugs. This argument has
been used, for example, to explain the consistent finding that
Black adolescents report lower drug use rates, both lifetime
and current, than their White counterparts. (However, other
plausible explanations exist. Some researchers, for example,
believe that Black and White adolescents display different
developmental patterns of drug use. White students tend to
experiment with drugs early, but turn away from drugs in late
adolescence as they prepare to enter college or the job mar-
ket. Blacks, by contrast, experiment later, often turning to drugs
when they find themselves unprepared for college or unable
to find a job.) Other students may actually overemphasize their
use of drugs, either because they do not take the survey seri-

ously, or simply to show off. One adolescent, for example, was heard to say just prior to taking our drug survey, "Well, let's see . . .What drugs should I say I'm using today?" Over-reporting actually appears to be more common than under-reporting.[5]

Yet despite these concerns, studies have shown that self-report data are, for the most part, valid.[6-9] Likewise, we have found that the results from our own self-report drug survey (described in the section, Comprehensive Drug Surveys) are so consistent across populations tested and year of administration that we are forced to conclude either the results are reliable or there is a "grand conspiracy" afoot.

The evidence for reliability notwithstanding, safeguards should be taken when administering self-report instruments. One strategy is to include an imaginary drug category in the survey. Alternatively, respondents can be asked directly to judge how accurate their responses were. An informal comparison of these two approaches by the present authors suggest that self-assessment of response accuracy is less effective than an imaginary drug item, perhaps for the same reasons that under- and over-reporting occur. Other secondary checks of reliability can also bolster our confidence in the self-report instrument. For instance, a *multiplicity technique* can be employed in which self-reports are compared with reports from other knowledgeable individuals.[10] Or, a *capture–recapture technique* can be utilized, which derives prevalence from the number of individuals initially identified who are subsequently "recaptured" in a second sample.[11]

Assessment Problems
Unique to Adolescents and Females

Owen and Nyberg[12] suggested the following common problems associated with assessment of drug use among adolescents:

1. Differentiating problematic alcohol/drug use from normal adolescent experimentation;
2. Differentiating abuse of alcohol/drugs from dependency;
3. Differentiating alcohol/drug problems from general behavioral problems, juvenile delinquency, or concomitant mental disorders; and
4. Expanding standardized assessment tools to measure drug use other than alcohol, because adolescents are more likely to present with drug problems than are adults. (Put more succinctly, adolescents today are *often polydrug users*.)

Owen and Nyberg added that terms frequently applied to adult users, such as "alcoholism" and "dependency," are themselves called into question when discussing adolescents because, as a group, they lack sufficient time or experience to achieve chronicity. We might add that the distinction between *licit* and *illicit* drugs must also be reexamined when applied to adolescents because of the statutory prohibitions against all drugs, except over-the-counter and physician-prescribed medications. As used throughout this article, licit and illicit will refer specifically to the legal status of specific drugs among adults.

When gender differences are factored into the assessment equation, another problem emerges. Because male adolescents typically report both more extensive and intensive use of both licit and illicit drugs, most instruments are designed around male use patterns. Yet when prevalence rates for substances used primarily by female adolescents (e.g., over-the-counter medications and wine coolers) are included, important gender differences appear. Other gender-specific issues requiring further clarification include:

1. Are adolescent females more or less truthful in their responses to questions about drug use than adolescent males?
2. Should drug use questions be worded differently for females than for males?

3. Does the testing situation (e.g., group vs individual interview) or the sex of the survey administrator have a gender effect?
4. Are there important interactions between gender and other related variables such as race, socioeconomic class, religion, or age?

Assessment Instruments

Clinical Assessment Instruments

In their 1983 article, Owen and Nyberg[12] reported findings from a survey of 70 adolescent treatment facilities across the United States concerning their assessment of adolescent drug use. They found that 78% of those facilities eliciting drug use data from their adolescent clients had developed their own in-house questionnaires. The instruments typically evolved informally and were integrated into the client interview. Although often reflecting the philosophy of the facility in which they were developed, such tests provide researchers and professionals at other agencies with little standardized information. Owen and Nyberg also found that, in many cases, the questionnaires employed were initially developed for adults and presented with little or no modification to adolescent clients. Among the more common instruments used to assess adolescent drug use among the facilities surveyed by Owen and Nyberg were: the MacAuliffe Inventory, WHO ME?, the Hystad Alcohol Use Profile, the Alibrandi Youth Diagnostic Screening Test, the Jellinek Chart, and the Heilman Chart.

Since the Owen and Nyberg review, a new wave of assessment instruments specifically applicable to adolescent populations have appeared. In 1991, a Center for Substance Abuse Treatment (CSAT) consensus panel reviewed current adolescent assessment instruments. The following is a description of those instruments reviewed by the panel that assess specifically for alcohol and other drug use. Further information on these and other related instruments can be found in a summary of the panel's conclusions by McLellan and Dembo.[13]

The Drug Use Screening Inventory (DUSI) is a multidimensional self-report instrument that has the important goal of "rationally and empirically" tying assessment to treatment. One-hundred and fifty yes/no items encompassing 10 specific domains are included in the first stage of a three-part assessment strategy. Vocabulary level for the DUSI is at or below the 6th grade, with an estimated age range for the instrument of 11–18 yr. Items are not gender specific and the instrument can be administered in a group or individual setting. Individual results on the DUSI are used to further evaluate selective domains of disturbance, and from there to target interventions based on evaluation findings. Tarter[14] and his group are currently engaged in a comprehensive program of standardizing their instrument and determining its clinical usefulness.

The Adolescent Drug Abuse Diagnosis (ADAD) is a 150-item instrument for structured interview administration with a format adopted from the Addiction Severity Index (ASI), an adult assessment instrument. The ADAD contains both alcohol- and other drug-related items, measuring:

1. The degree to which the client has had difficulty with each type of drug-related problem;
2. The interviewer's ratings of the client's need for treatment in each problem area;
3. The degree of the client's desire and motivation for treatment; and
4. The degree of the client's denial or misrepresentation of his/her situation and behavior.

The instrument is administered by a trained interviewer and takes 55 min to complete and score. A comprehensive evaluation of the client is provided that includes 10-point severity ratings for each of nine life problem areas. Composite scores measuring the client's behavioral change in each problem area during and after treatment can also be calculated. A short version (83 items) is also available for followup, evaluation, and assessment of treatment outcomes.

The Personal Experience Inventory (PEI) is a comprehensive adolescent assessment instrument consisting of several parts. Part I, the Chemical Involvement Problem Severity (CIPS), provides extensive coverage of alcohol and other drug use and abuse and related problems. Part II consists of a Psychosocial Section (PS) that assesses personal risk and adjustment, family and peer environmental risk, eating disorders, sexual and physical abuse, suicide risk, and psychiatric referral. Because the PEI does not provide the basis for a *DSM–III–R*[15] diagnosis, the Adolescent Diagnostic Interview that is available with the PEI should also be used. Part III of the instrument is the Personal Experience Screening Questionnaire (PESQ), which consists of a 38-item questionnaire that screens specifically for alcohol and other drug problems. The purpose of the PEI battery is:

1. To assess the involvement of psychological and behavioral issues in alcohol and drug problems;
2. To assess psychological risk factors believed to be associated with teenage chemical involvement;
3. To evaluate response bias or invalid responding;
4. To screen for the presence of problems other than substance abuse, such as school or family problems; and
5. To aid in determining the appropriateness of inpatient or outpatient addiction treatment.

The PEI is self-administered and is written at a sixth-grade reading level. According to the author the scales appear to be reliable and valid for Whites, Blacks, Native Americans, and Hispanics.

The Assessment of Chemical Health Inventory (ACHI) was developed to assess the nature and extent of substance abuse and associated psychosocial problems, and develop a standard that will facilitate communication among treatment providers. Although the 128-item self-administered instrument contains alcohol- and other drug-related items, it does not provide quantitative data on frequency or duration of use for specific illicit drugs. However, the ACHI does provide scores on degree of need for use of drugs, on reasons for use, and on consequences of use. It also contains critical life items (family estrangement, social impact, depression, family support, family chemical use, self-regard/abuse, and physical and/or sexual abuse) that indicate the adolescent's need for immediate attention. The ACHI takes 15–20 min to complete and is at a sixth-grade reading level. It does not differentiate by gender.

The Prevention Intervention Management and Evaluation System (PMES) is a 150-item instrument that can be used to:

1. Assess substance abuse and other life problems;
2. Assist in planning treatment; and
3. Provide followup assessment and evaluation data on treatment outcomes.

The PMES contains a Client Intake Form with questions on demographics, referral source and process, socioeconomic and family background, school problems, legal status, alcohol/drug use history, and a checklist to determine areas in most need of attention. An information form on Family, Friends, and Self contains Family Relations, Peer Activity, and Self Scales, with each scale measuring areas of need in its respective domain. The PMES assumes a sixth-grade reading level and takes 1 h to complete. An individual score can also be calculated that may be compared to scores obtained by a normative sample. Although promising, the instrument has not yet been studied sufficiently to determine its psychometric fitness.

The Problem Oriented Screening Instrument for Teenagers (POSIT) is a self-administered 128-item questionnaire designed for use by male and female adolescents age 12–19. It is an initial screening tool used to identify potential problem areas that require further assessment. This instrument is not intended as a measure of change or outcome. Following initial screening with the POSIT, a more thorough assessment tool (e.g., the PEI for alcohol and other drug use) is administered. Some questions are age related in that they are scored only for adolescents over 16. Other items are age-specific and handled differently in scoring. The POSIT screens for 10 problem areas: alcohol/other drug use, physical and mental health, family and peer relations, educational and vocational status, social skills, leisure/recreation, and aggressive behavior. It is brief and easy to use and is written on a sixth-grade reading level. The POSIT is available in both Spanish and English.

The Substance Abuse Subtle Screening Inventory (SASSI), although not reviewed by the CSAT Consensus Panel, deserves mention here because it includes both adolescent male and female versions. The SASSI is a one page (both sides) test that requires about 12 min to administer and score. Psychometric studies have demonstrated over 90% accuracy with high retest reliability for substance abuse screening. Eight subscales provide a range of clinical information, including a screening for denial and codependency. The instrument has been cross-validated with random participants, including minority and ethnic groups.[16]

Comprehensive Drug Surveys

Although the instruments reviewed are designed for use in specific client-centered settings, prevalence data used to establish baselines and effect policy decisions are typically derived from broader-based general surveys of substance use. Here we review three such instruments. The first two are widely recognized national surveys. The third is our own drug survey, which provides the basis for much of the discussion of gender differences in drug use that follows.

The Michigan Study

This survey is the cornerstone of an ongoing national research and reporting program entitled "Monitoring the Future: A Continuing Study of Lifestyles and Values of Youth." Administered each year since 1975 by the University of Michigan's Institute for Social Research and sponsored by the National Institute on Drug Abuse (NIDA), the instrument is based on a representative sample of seniors in public and private high schools in the contiguous United States. Also included are followup data from previous graduating classes and, since 1980, representative samples of American college students. In 1991 the survey was expanded to include 8th and 10th grade students.

The Michigan Study provides the most comprehensive information available on national trends for lifetime and current drug use among older adolescents. It also reports data on grade of first use, trends in use at lower grade levels, intensity of drug use, attitudes and beliefs concerning types of drug use, and students' perceptions of relevant aspects of the social environment.[17] One weakness of the Michigan study should also be mentioned. The survey's emphasis on high school seniors has, in the past, neglected the ontogeny of drug use during the early adolescent years. In fact, we provide data suggesting that both experimentation and current drug use may actually decline in the senior year, at least among females. This problem has recently been addressed with the addition 8th and 10th graders into the study in 1991. Yet the critical time for initiation into drug use appears to be even earlier, between the 6th and 8th grades, which is still outside the range of the Michigan Study.

The National Household Survey on Drug Use

Conducted biannually since 1971, the survey is based on household interviews with individuals 12 and older (the interview format differentiates it from the other two surveys reviewed in this section). Although emphasizing intact families, the National Household Survey under-represents many of the family configurations prevalent in today's society. Moreover, drug use estimates for specific subgroups are sometimes based on modest to small sample sizes, which may lead to substantial sampling error.[18]

The Duval Survey

Since 1988, the Duval Survey has been administered annually to 6th, 8th, 10th, and 12th graders throughout the state of Florida. To date, nearly 100,000 students in nine Florida counties have participated in the project (the majority coming from a single large school district in Northeast Florida). For the past 4 yr, the survey format has been standardized to provide information concerning long-term changes in drug use and attitudes. Students are asked about their lifetime and current (30-d) use across 18 drug categories. Attitudes toward drug use are also sampled, as are style of use (experimental, recreational, regular, dependent, or other), place of use, drug sources, and perceived change in personal drug use over the past 12 mo. The Duval Survey contains gender-specific drug categories, including smokeless tobacco and steroids for males and over-the-counter drugs (OTCs) and wine coolers for females.

Truthfulness and care in responding are routinely assessed during administration, scoring, and analysis of the Duval Survey. Among the safeguards are an imaginary drug category (for truthfulness of responding) and a crosscheck of certain demographic items (for accuracy of responding). Data from participants flagged during the validity checks are excluded from further analyses.[19]

Gender Differences in Adolescent Drug Use

We now turn to the findings derived from the instruments reviewed in the previous section, particularly those from the comprehensive drug surveys. One consistent difference between male and female adolescents is that female adolescents use fewer drugs and take them less frequently than males. Johnston et al.[17] reported, for example, that "daily use [of alcohol] is reported by 5.3% of the senior males vs. only 1.6% of the senior females [in their 1991 survey]. Also, males are more likely than females to drink larger quantities of alcohol in a single sitting; 38% of senior males report taking five or more drinks in a row in the prior two weeks vs. 21% of senior females. These sex differences are observable [among 8th and 10th graders as well]" (p. 55). The data are tempered, however, by other findings. First, if marijuana is considered the threshold between so-called "gateway" drugs (e.g., alcohol and tobacco) and more dangerous drugs, than almost equal numbers of males and females (13 vs 11%) pass that threshold at least once a year. Second, females actually report having tried certain types of drugs significantly more often than males.

Lifetime Use Rates
for Adolescent Males and Females

In Fig. 1, lifetime use rates for male and female adolescents across 17 drug categories are presented. These data represent the combined results for all 6th, 8th, 10th, and 12th graders who took the Duval Survey between 1990 and 1993 (a total of 64,919 participants). The stability of results across the four yearly surveys allows us to collapse the data across this variable without effect. The same consistency is seen across the nine counties represented in the data, with one exception: Lifetime use rates for smokeless tobacco were significantly higher among students from rural counties as compared to use rates among students residing in the single large metropolitan district included in the survey. For example, in 1992 the reported lifetime use rates for both males and females across the rural counties ranged from 28–31%; for the metropolitan sample from the same year the prevalence was only 15%.

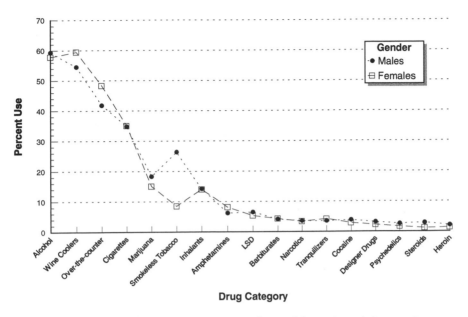

Fig. 1. Lifetime drug use among male and female adolescents.

Although reported lifetime use rates are essentially the same for most drug categories, several important gender differences can be seen in Fig. 1. Among the drugs of choice, males tend to experiment more often with smokeless tobacco and, to a lesser extent, with marijuana. Still, reported use rates by female adolescents are considerable for both drug categories. Some will find it surprising that 9% of all females reported trying smokeless tobacco. However, this figure is in line with data provided by Riley et al.[20] who studied smokeless tobacco use among 5683 teenage females in four southeastern states. The average age of the respondents was 16 yr, with major urban areas specifically excluded. The researchers found that 15.3% of all female respondents had tried smokeless tobacco, with an average age of initial use of 13.56 yr. Approximately 3–4% of the sample were regular users. Although experimentation with smokeless tobacco by males is closely associated with use of other drugs, modeling effects are more important among females. Moreover, perceived negative consequences among White females, modeling influences among Native American females, and use of other substances among Black females were the best predictors of level of use. Riley et al. argued that, "Taken together, these results provide a strong argument for beginning prevention programs in elementary school, prior to the period when most children try smokeless tobacco" (p. 217). Among the illicit drugs, males report steroid use twice as often as females (2.83% vs 1.07%), although the total number of respondents is too small to assure meaningful comparisons.

For their part, females report substantially greater use of wine coolers than males. They also report greater experimentation with psychoactive drugs. These include both nonprescription OTCs and their prescription counterparts (amphetamines, barbiturates, and tranquilizers). Psychoactive drugs are "mood-altering" substances, sometimes called "uppers" and "downers." They provide a means for regulating activity level to cope with pressures of daily living, such as staying awake to study for a big examination and getting to sleep after a particularly stressful day. Females may be more disposed to use these drugs than males are for at least two reasons: First, adolescent girls, in particular, may use nonprescription diet pills and their prescription counterparts, amphetamines, specifically for weight control. Second, these drugs, particularly the barbiturates and tranquilizers, are more commonly prescribed for adult females than for adult males. This difference is directly related to the greater percentage of females diagnosed with depression, anxiety, and related mental health disorders. According to Greenspan,[21] women comprise almost two-thirds of the adult population found in general psychiatric, community mental health, and outpatient psychiatric facilities. Whether females are more susceptible to disorders of mood is unclear; still the fact remains that women do report stress in many areas of their lives.[22,23] To deal with their stressors, they may turn to mood altering medications, often in conjunction with alcohol.

Based on the relationship between mood altering drugs and adult females, adolescent females may also be placed at risk as follows:

1. They may have better access than males to mood altering drugs through their mothers;
2. They may find in their mothers a role model who predisposes them to earlier and more sustained use; and
3. They may face issues of growing up female that produce unique stressors in their lives that lead to the use of certain classes of drugs.

Cohort Trends

Table 1 provides a summary of reported lifetime and current (30-d) drug use rates among adolescent females. These data represent 30,109 students (Grades 6, 8, 10, and 12) from a single urban school district who participated in the Duval Survey between 1990 and 1993. The substances included in Table 1 are both adolescent drugs of choice and drugs used extensively by females. Going down the columns provides a summary of the percent of females at each grade level who experimented with, or were currently using, a particular drug in a given year. Moving across rows gives information on changes in use rates for each grade level over the past 4 yr. Most important, two cohort groups at each grade level have now participated in one test–retest cycle. The prevalencies by grade for each pair have been averaged and then compared with their average results 2 yr later. These comparisons are read diagonally. The difference in the average scores across a 2-yr test–retest cycle is given under "Proportion Change." To take an example, the prevalencies for lifetime cigaret use among 6th graders assessed in 1990 and 1991 were .22 and .18, respectively. These same cohorts were retested in 1992

Table 1
Cohort Trends Among Female Adolescents

Drug/grade	Lifetime use by year					Current use by year				
	1990	1991	1992	1993	Proportion change	1990	1991	1992	1993	Proportion change
Cigaret										
6th	**.22**	**.18**	.20	.19		**.31**	**.32**	.32	.35	
8th	.39	.38	**.43**	**.38**	**.22**	.45	.40	**.42**	**.45**	**.13**
10th	**.47**	**.43**	.49	.48	.10	**.42**	**.40**	.42	.45	.01
12th	.45	.41	**.48**	**.46**	**.02**	.48	.39	**.42**	**.44**	**.02**
Alcohol										
6th	**.37**	**.38**	.31	.32		**.45**	**.45**	.48	.47	
8th	.59	.62	**.64**	**.59**	**.23**	.55	.56	**.58**	**.59**	**.14**
10th	**.74**	**.73**	.76	.75	.14	**.57**	**.58**	.58	.61	.04
12th	.79	.77	**.80**	**.78**	**.05**	.65	.53	**.55**	**.54**	**-.04**
Wine coolers										
6th	**.40**	**.40**	.37	.37		**.49**	**.46**	.47	.46	
8th	.63	.66	**.65**	**.62**	**.23**	.53	.52	**.53**	**.54**	**.06**
10th	**.74**	**.73**	.74	.72	.09	**.47**	**.49**	.46	.50	-.04
12th	.79	.77	**.77**	**.76**	**-.03**	.48	.46	**.43**	**.42**	**-.06**
Marijuana										
6th	**.04**	**.03**	.04	.04		**.46**	**.42**	.47	.46	
8th	.15	.13	**.15**	**.14**	**.10**	.57	.56	**.59**	**.60**	**.15**
10th	**.26**	**.23**	.24	.26	.11	**.49**	**.57**	.60	.54	.00
12th	.35	.26	**.28**	**.27**	**.03**	.46	.43	**.46**	**.51**	**-.05**

OTC									
6th	**.40**	**.41**	.37	.38		**.72**	**.80**	.77	.77	
8th	.50	.54	**.52**	**.50**	**.10**	.78	.83	**.79**	**.84**	**.06**
10th	**.55**	**.50**	.48	.59	.02	**.75**	**.77**	.76	.79	−.03
12th	.53	.53	**.50**	**.50**	**−.05**	.68	.74	**.69**	**.74**	**−.04**
Amphetamines									
6th	**.03**	**.03**	.04	.04		**.66**	**.63**	.65	.65	
8th	.09	.09	**.10**	**.09**	**.06**	.62	.62	**.59**	**.69**	**.00**
10th	**.12**	**.12**	.14	.14	.05	**.48**	**.46**	.60	.48	−.08
12th	.10	.09	**.10**	**.12**	**−.01**	.32	.40	**.40**	**.44**	**−.05**
Barbiturates									
6th	**.02**	**.02**	.03	.03		**.59**	**.63**	.56	.75	
8th	.04	.05	**.06**	**.05**	**.03**	.63	.75	**.66**	**.74**	**.09**
10th	**.06**	**.05**	.07	.08	.02	**.55**	**.53**	.56	.60	−.10
12th	.04	.04	**.05**	**.06**	**−.01**	.48	.48	**.58**	**.47**	**−.02**
Tranquilizers									
6th	**.03**	**.01**	.03	.03		**.60**	**.73**	.57	.47	
8th	.04	.04	**.04**	**.04**	**.02**	.66	.54	**.59**	**.56**	**−.08**
10th	**.07**	**.05**	.05	.07	.02	**.44**	**.49**	.48	.58	−.06
12th	.06	.06	**.06**	**.05**	**.00**	.39	.38	**.61**	**.35**	**.03**

and 1993, when their prevalence rates were .43 and .38, respectively. When the average prevalency rates for the two 6th grade groups are compared with their average results 2 yr later, a .22 increase is seen.

These data should by no means be construed as longitudinal, because many original students did not participate in the retest, whereas other new students entered the population in the interim. Moreover, those individuals who were not retested probably represent a select group comprised of a high percentage of high school dropouts. Still, the cohort comparisons do provide important trend information.

Looking first across rows, we see that lifetime use of specific substances has remained relatively stable among adolescent females for the past 4 yr. This is particularly true of the prescription psychoactives. OTCs, however, have shown a modest (1–4%) decline across the four grade levels during this period. (Percent declines reported here and elsewhere in this section are calculated by subtracting the average use rates for 1991–1992 from the average use rates for 1993–1994.) There is also an indication that experimentation with alcoholic beverages, and more specifically wine coolers, is declining among 6th graders (6% for alcohol of all types). Of particular interest is the fact that reported experimentation with wine coolers is actually higher than for alcohol use among 6th and 8th graders. This supports a finding by Barton and Johnson[24] that many of the so-called "gateway" substances are not perceived as drugs at all by children and adolescents and suggests that more emphasis should be given to educating young adolescents about the dangers of substances that may otherwise be legal for adults. Finally, lifetime marijuana use has seen a modest decline (3%) among high school seniors, whereas smoking has shown a 1–4% increase across grades.

Yearly changes in current use rates for the drugs examined in Table 1 display somewhat more variability than the lifetime rates. Generally speaking, among female adolescents who report having tried a particular drug, approx 50% indicate that they have used it in the past 30 d. (The current use rates reported for the Duval Survey tend to be somewhat higher than those reported in other surveys because only those students who indicate they have tried a drug are then asked whether they have used in the last month. Most other instruments calculate current use as a proportion of the total sample.) The greatest change is seen among 6th grade marijuana users, who report a 15% increase in current use over the past 2 yr as compared to the previous 2 yr. This increase has occurred despite the fact that lifetime use has remained constant. Other large increases in current use are seen for amphetamine use among 10th and 12th graders (7% each), barbiturate use among 6th graders (6%), and tranquilizer use among 10th and 12th graders (8 and 10%, respectively). On the downturn are tranquilizer use among 6th graders (−13%) and alcohol use among 12th graders (−6%).

Cohort changes over a 2-yr period are summarized in Table 1 under "Proportion change." One obvious conclusion drawn from even the most cursory glance at this column is that the critical time for initiation into drug use is between the 6th and 8th grades. Over this period there is a 22% increase in experimentation with cigarets, a 23% increase in experimentation with alcohol, and, more specifically, wine coolers, and a 10% increase in experimentation with marijuana and OTCs. Substantial increases in lifetime use continue into the 10th grade for alcohol (14%), marijuana (11%), cigarets (10%), and wine coolers (9%). Thus, the pattern that emerges from the data in Table 1 is that experimentation with drugs peaks between the 6th and 8th grades, continues to increase but at a slower rate between the 8th and 10th grades, and shows almost no increase in the 12th grade.

One disparate finding should be noted. Declines in lifetime use rates appear in several instances. In true cohort data these declines would not occur. We offer two explanations for these discrepancies: First, we suspect that some portion of the declines, seen only among 12th graders, is owing to forgetfulness. That is, although most adolescents probably recall something about their first drink or first cigaret (and, in fact, may still be engaged in their use), they may not remember purchasing a box of NoDoz several years ago. Second, we have already alluded to the principle weakness of the trend data reported in Table 1, viz., that losses from the student pool between testings involve a substantial, but undetermined, number of high school dropouts. To the extent that these students are over-represented among early experimenters, their loss from the sample should result in a decline in lifetime prevalence rates.

Current (30-d) use data generally parallel those for lifetime use among the gateway substances, with the critical period occurring between the 6th and 8th grades. During this interval, current use of marijuana increased 15%, use of alcohol increased 14%, and use of cigarets increased 13%. The increase in prevalency for wine coolers during the same period was more moderate (7%), perhaps indicating that current use of alcohol is more closely associated with forms of liquor other than wine coolers. In this regard, the suggestion of Johnston et al.[17] that female adolescents often date older boys who are more likely to turn to beer and hard liquor than to wine coolers, must be considered. Other researchers have also identified the preadolescent period as a time of particular risk for initiation into regular drug use. For example, the Centers for Disease Control recently found that, although only 1% of all 12 yr olds reported smoking the previous week, 12% of the 15 yr olds and 25% of the 18 yr olds surveyed identified themselves as current smokers. The declines in current use rates seen for some drugs in Table 1 reflect a combination of systematic loss of at-risk students across grade levels as well as real declines in current use among older students. However, the contribution of each has yet to be determined.

Predisposing Factors

A consideration of the individual "risk factors" involved in adolescent drug use is prerequisite to the application of specific prevention or treatment strategies. However, before discussing gender, or any other factor predisposing drug use, we must first distinguish between *causal* variables and *carrier* variables. In the social sciences, a causal variable is one that, when manipulated, has a direct effect on behavior. In a well-designed experimental study, a variable thought to influence behavior is manipulated under controlled conditions and its effects noted. Only in this manner can causal relationships be determined. A carrier variable, by contrast, is not a causal agent. Rather, as the name implies, it merely "carries" causal factors with it, much as a river carries objects along its course. Research designs that classify participants using carrier variables are termed *descriptive*. Descriptive studies, although an important first step in organizing the data in any science, provide no direct evidence of cause and effect. Gender is a carrier variable. Therefore, studies that merely observe differences among males and female participants (and this includes most of the research on gender differences among substance users) are descriptive in nature. That is, they provide correlational, not causative, information. Other carrier variables include age, race, and socioeconomic class. With this distinction in mind, let us turn now to some of the prominent variables included in the "at-risk" category.

Males and females share many risk factors for substance abuse. In this section, however, we focus on factors unique to substance-abusing or addicted women, and to those common factors that appear to produce differential outcomes in males and females. This approach is supported by growing evidence that significant differences exist between chemically addicted men and women, and that these differences may be discovered through careful study of early life experiences and subsequent drinking and drug taking behaviors.[23,25] For example, a higher percentage of female than male alcoholics use drugs other than, or in addition to, alcohol.[22,26] Likewise, psychoactive drugs are prescribed more frequently for women than for men, and the possibility of cross-addiction is consequently higher.[23,27] And because they metabolize alcohol differently than men, women may be more susceptible to its adverse effects (*see* Biological Factors).[28] Women also progress more quickly than men, and perhaps follow a different developmental course, as they move from heavy to problematic drug use.

In addition, we would argue that risk factors have always been differentiated on the basis of gender and that, until recently, the factors examined were those most closely associated with male substance use. That is to say, substance abuse is still seen as primarily a male problem. This remains the case despite over a decade of research demonstrating that one in three alcoholics and two in five drug abusers in this country are women.[29–31] Even professionals tend to underestimate the seriousness of alcoholism and drug abuse among females.[32,33] When they are identified, chemically dependent females are less likely to enter appropriate treatment programs than males.[31] These findings give us every reason to believe that a moral stigma against female substance abusers still exists.[22]

Sex Role Conflict

Conflict over sex roles is one source of stress faced by women today. Whereas some women drink, use drugs, or both in response to stress associated with narrow and confining roles, the change in traditional sex roles has also been accompanied by greater occupational stress and demands of multiple conflicting role expectations.[22,23,25,27,34] Several researchers, including pioneer Sharon Wilsnack, hypothesize that rather than womanhood acting as a shield against the development of drinking problems, the traditional female role with its restricted behavioral norms, options, and expectations actually generates psychic sex role conflicts that many women seek to subdue through the abuse of alcohol and other drugs.[25,35]

Wilsnack's preliminary research suggests that women who experience conflict between a conscious identity with masculine attitudes and feelings drink and use drugs to feel more feminine. Later studies support the sex role conflict theory and also demonstrate an opposite pattern of sex role conflict often seen in younger alcohol/other drug abusers: conscious rejection of the female role and an unconscious need to meet society's norms of womanhood.[25] Both types of chemically dependent women, those who reject and those who accept their culturally given identity, abuse drugs for the same underlying motive—to relieve psychic conflict.

Parents

Parents are known to play a central role in deviant behavior in general, and drug use in particular.[36,37] The reason is simple: Causal variables associated with substance use arise from two sources—*nature,* the genetic predisposition of the individual, and *nurture,* the environment to which the individual is exposed. *Parents provide both.* Research on parental influences has focused on three main areas: parental use of drugs, parental attitudes toward drug use, and parent–child interaction.

The first two issues—parental drug use and parental attitudes toward drugs—stem from the parents' role as teachers. Prior to adolescence parents are powerful role models for the child, shaping both behavior and attitudes. We should not be surprised, then, to find that greater than 65% of abusing adolescent females come from families where one or both parents are alcohol or other drug abusers.[38] A common family configuration for the female substance abuser consists of a dominant mother and alcoholic father. Developmentally, the critical period for parental influence is thought to be between the ages of 4 and 9 yr. As discussed later, by adolescence the parents' influence has begun to wane as it is replaced by peer group norms. This seems particularly true for drug use.

Parent–child interaction, the third issue, is multifaceted, leaving a thorough discussion well beyond the scope of this chapter. However, it can be said that chemically addicted females have more disturbed family backgrounds than do men.[39,40] Addicted females are also more likely than men to be the victims of child abuse or neglect, including sexual abuse and incest.[32] Psychologically, parental–child interaction has been linked to identity crises; poor, inadequate, or distorted self-images; low self-esteem; and a poor self-concept.[22,25,35] Addiction is a cyclic disorder that can be seen in generational family systems. In addition to issues of control, mothers who abuse chemicals model negative coping strategies for their daughters. According to Fejes-Mendoza,[41] the substance-abusing female often uses drugs as a means of dealing with persistent exposure to violence, including physical abuse and rape.

Relationships

Adolescent females are similar to adult women in their assessment of relationships, inasmuch as they often do not distinguish between love and codependency. In many families, young women have received reinforcement for acting out codependency characteristics.[42] Frequently, adolescent females and their adult counterparts become involved with addicted or abusive men. These dysfunctional love relationships can heighten drug abuse, thwart treatment, and predispose relapse.[43-45]

Personality Traits

Jessor's group has noted that, at least for marijuana use, personality factors are more predictive of adolescent involvement than is true for college-age students.[46] Kandel[47] identified rebelliousness, acceptance of nontraditional values, and lack of conventionality as characteristics of substance users. Other correlates to drug use include creativity, need for new and varied experiences, risk taking, radical political views, political dissension, and lower commitment to religion.

Although it is easy to see how the personality factors just described may well lead an adolescent to experiment with drugs, we should not forget that the same factors are also important concomitants to adequate identity formation. Adolescence provides a unique opportunity for young women on the cusp of adulthood to try out different roles, lifestyles, and behaviors before settling on the one identity that fits them best. In fact, society intuitively honors and encourages this experimentation through what Erikson[48] called a *moratorium,* a slackening of the rules during adolescence so that various options can be perused. The crucial question, then, is: When does normal and necessary experimentation become abnormal, harmful, and addicting? It is in this context, we believe, that research concerned with identifying a threshold for deviancy becomes important based on the sheer number of deviant acts and/or the commission of a particular act that marks the transition from normal adolescent experimentation to serious deviancy (*see* Robins and Wish[49] for one attempt to compare these two criteria).

Psychologically, female substance users:

1. Attempted suicide more often than males;[50,51]
2. Are prone to eating disorders;[52] and
3. Are apt to be hospitalized for mental disorders.[32]

Central to much of the research pertaining to psychological risk factors is the belief that drug use represents a coping strategy for dealing with life problems. This perspective explains why disruptive early life experiences and losses appear to be more prevalent among female substance abusers than in male abusers.[53,54] Female users are more likely than males to come from families with histories of substance abuse, criminality, and mental illness.[50] Additionally, over 90% have dropped out of school and greater than 75% have been exposed to violent situations.[38]

In studying therapeutic communities, Jainchill et al.[55] found that female addicts have more psychiatric diagnoses than male addicts. Others have noted depression to be paramount among female substance abusers who entered treatment.[56,57] Mooney[42] argued that a common dual diagnoses for adolescent females is: depression; suicide; self-destructive behavior; cyclothymic disorder; and narcissistic, histrionic, or dependent personality disorders.

Finally, the female adolescent's general orientation toward the future and goal-directed behavior may affect drug use, as suggested by Johnston et al.[17] They reported that students who indicate they are probably or definitely "college-bound" have lower rates of illicit drug use than those who indicate they probably or definitely are not going to continue their education. These researchers add that, "For any given drug, the differences between these two self-identified groups of students tend to be greatest in the eighth grade. This could reflect an earlier age of onset for the noncollege-bound, and/ or the fact that they are a more select subgroup in the earlier grades" (p. 55).

Social Networks

Beginning in preadolescence (ages 10–12), parental influence begins to wane as peer influence increases. This is particularly true in the area of drug involvement.[58,59] Parents are not, however, completely excluded from the adolescent's life. In general, "Parental influences are stronger for issues related to future roles; peer influences are stronger for issues related to immediate adolescent life styles" (p. 257).[3]

Erikson[48] argued convincingly that peer groups provide the young adolescent with a *pseudoidentity* as he or she deliberately casts aside the values, beliefs, and attitudes instilled by the parents in order to achieve the distance and perspective necessary to evaluate who he/she is as an individual and eventually to form a sense of personal identity. This view explains the gradual increase in peer group influence between pre- and midadolescence and the concomitant decline in parental influence. It also explains the fact that after peaking at about the 9th grade, peer group influence gradually declines as it is replaced by the adolescent's burgeoning confidence in his or her own sense of self.[60] Regarding prevention, Erikson's theory suggests that an adequate measure of identity formation might not only furnish insight into the adolescent's developmental status, but also provide clues as to the most effective type of prevention message—parent based, peer based, or identity based.

Three other characteristics of peer influence on adolescent drug use are important to note: First, researchers have found that association with users of a particular drug is the best predictor of subsequent use by the adolescent.[59,61] However, this statement will ultimately need to be modified to include the status of the adolescent's identity development. It seems likely that a youth with a well-developed sense of self will be less susceptible to the influence of others than will one who is in the early stages of identity formation. Second, peer influences appear to be transient. That is, the predictive value of drug use within a peer group is immediate and short-lived. Although this finding is in line with the concept of a temporary pseudoidentity in early adolescence, it also appears true of older adolescents and college students.[62] Third, females may be more susceptible to peer influence than males.[46,63] However, this issue is not yet settled. Berndt[59] found that boys conform more than girls to peer influences when antisocial behavior is involved, whereas others suggest that boys and girls may be equally disposed toward peer influence, but girls are less likely to participate with peers in antisocial behavior.[64,65]

Biological Factors

Women appear to be physiologically different from men in the way their bodies react to drugs. To indicate the direction research in this area is developing, we describe two commonly found sex differences related specifically to alcohol consumption and their possible physiological correlates, as reported by Gordis.[29]

First, women become intoxicated more quickly than men. One explanation is that, because women's bodies have a lower total water content than men's bodies of comparable size, alcohol may become less diluted in women when it diffuses into intra- and intercellular fluids. Another possibility is that more alcohol is metabolized in the stomachs of men than of women, specifically by the enzyme alcohol dehydrogenase. This leaves less alcohol available for general circulation throughout the body. Frezza et al.[66] reported that such "first-pass metabolism" is virtually nonexistent in alcoholic females. Finally, hormonal fluctuations during the menstrual cycle may affect the rate of alcohol metabolism in females. For example, research has shown that premenstrual syndrome (PMS) and abstinence syndrome share common symptomatology and can trigger initial use as well as possible relapse.[67] However, the direction of cause and effect is presently unclear, as seen in a study by Wilsnack et al.[68] where dysmenorrhea (menstrual discomfort, heavy bleeding and irregularity) was found associated with chronic heavy drinking.

Second, chronic alcohol abuse takes a greater toll on women's bodies than on men's. Female alcoholics have a death rate 50–100% higher than male alcoholics. Women die after a shorter period of use and from lower consumption levels than do men. Women, more than men, are vulnerable to liver disease secondary to alcohol consumption; they may also increase their risk of breast cancer and infertility. The reasons behind this heightened susceptibility remain to be discovered.

Theoretical Orientations

Finally, we turn our attention from individual risk factors to theoretical approaches that attempt to integrate our knowledge about the precursors of substance use. As yet no one theory has succeeded in adequately integrating the many factors associated with adolescent drug use. However, preliminary steps toward a more comprehensive understanding of the problem have been taken. In this section we describe briefly four theoretical orientations. A word of caution, however. We believe it unlikely that one particular theory will allow us to adequately explain all the social, psychological, and biological variables involved in substance abuse. Rather, the reader should think in terms of meta-integration, that is, an integration and informed selection of the theories themselves based on the specific problems at hand.

Operant Theory

Primarily an outgrowth of the work of Skinner,[69] operant approaches to behavior analysis have their origin in the ancient philosophical tradition of *hedonism*. Hedonists believe that an individual will do whatever necessary to maximize pleasure and minimize pain. Operant theories merely define pleasure and pain more precisely. Pleasure becomes a *reinforcer* (less technically, a "reward"), any consequence that increases the frequency of the behavior it follows. Pain becomes a *pun-*

isher (or "aversive stimulus"), any consequence that decreases the frequency of the behavior it follows. A radical interpretation of operant conditioning suggests that all human behavior results from, i.e., is controlled by, its consequences.

Operant theory has been applied to substance use by Akers[70] and Burgess and Akers.[71] Akers et al.[72] suggested that "Whether deviant or conforming behavior is acquired or persists depends on past and present rewards or punishments for the behavior and the rewards and punishments attached to alternative behavior—*differential reinforcement. . . .*" (p. 838). Differential reinforcement is an operant concept that is often overlooked when attempts are made to alter a child's behavior. Punishing inappropriate behavior often fails because no adequately reinforced alternatives are provided. That is, it is never enough to say "Don't do that." Instead, the child should be told, "Don't do that, *do this instead,*" while a rewarding alternative behavior is presented. Aker's theory also emphasizes the social nature of many of the reinforcers affecting drug use behavior: "[In acquiring norms, attitudes and orientations,] the principle behavior effects come from interaction in or under the influence of those *groups which control individuals' major sources of reinforcement and punishment and expose them to behavioral models and normative definitions*)" (p. 838, italics in the original). As for gender differences in drug use, operant theory holds out the possibility that the environment reinforces and punishes female drug use behavior in ways that are quite different from what males experience.

Social Learning Theory

Social learning theory represents a general psychological approach to behavior change that has proven to be a fertile source of concepts relevant to an understanding of substance use. The most influential theoretician behind this approach is

Albert Bandura.[73] He and others make a clear distinction between *learning* a particular behavior and *performing* that behavior. Learning is an automatic process that occurs when an individual observes a model perform (and for this reason the outcome is often referred to as *observational learning*). Because information conveyed by the model is processed automatically, the trick is to get the learner to observe what the model is doing. A number of variables have been shown to be effective in making the model (for better or worse) more effectual, three of which have particular relevance to substance abuse:

1. *Perceived similarity*—the more like oneself the observer perceives the model to be, the more influential the model becomes;
2. *Inherent properties*—the more novel and salient the model, the more effective he/she becomes; and
3. *Power*—the possession of something the observer wants and/or fears and the ability and willingness to share it with the observer makes the model more effective.

Knowledge acquired through observation is retained in memory and may serve as the basis for performance at a later time. Performance consists of an imitative response based on stored information about the model's behavior. However, whether the observer actually carries out the learned behavior depends on the environmental contingencies of reward and punishment. That is, although learning is primarily cognitive, performance is a function of operant conditioning. To take a relevant example, almost everyone in our society knows how to hold and fire a gun—not necessarily by actually having pulled a trigger, but simply by seeing the behavior modeled repeatedly on television and in the movies. Fortunately, however, most of us will never perform this behavior, although we could certainly do so, because of the punishing consequences that would likely follow. This leads to another central concept of social learning theory, *vicarious* reinforcement and punishment. A person need not fire a gun at someone to determine what the environmental consequences will be. Instead, information about the consequences that accrue to the model is stored away as part of the learning process. If we observe that the model's behavior is rewarded, we ourselves will be more likely to imitate that behavior; conversely, if we see that the model is punished for his or her actions, we will be less likely to perform similarly.

This brief account of social learning theory leaves out much of the richness of Bandura's[73] model. However, it does provide enough information for us to examine briefly one model of substance use based on observational learning. Kandel's[3] "adolescent socialization theory" focuses on the interactions among adolescents, peers, and parents. She suggested that central to an understanding of adolescent behavior is "the extent to which the behaviors of adolescents are dependent upon the intragenerational influences of peers, or the intergenerational influences of adults, especially parents" (p. 256). One way peers and adults exert their influence is through the behaviors they model. Kandel suggested the two processes involved:

> The first is imitation, in which youths model their own behaviors or attitudes on other's behaviors by simply observing and replicating the behaviors or, in the case of parental drug behaviors, transposing them into forms more acceptable to the youth's lifestyle. . . . The second process is social reinforcement: Adolescents internalize definitions and exhibit behaviors and values approved by significant others. (p. 256)

As noted earlier, Kandel found that parental and peer influences are issue-specific. Whereas parents retain influence in the sphere of future plans and goals, peers exercise preeminent leverage in the realm of immediate lifestyle.

Developmental Theories

Recently, theories have emerged that take the child's developmental status into account. Russac and Weaver[74] argued that substance abuse professionals must move away from a quantitative approach to prevention and treatment, one where all children are viewed as basically the same, and toward a more qualitative approach that views childhood as a series of developmental stages, each with its own unique characteristics. The implication for prevention and treatment professionals who adopt a qualitative perspective is that no single prevention message or intervention strategy can be applied to all client populations simply by modulating its level of difficulty for presentation to individuals of varying age groups and educational backgrounds. Intervention is conceived, instead, in terms of messages, instructional techniques, evaluation tools, and treatment strategies designed for children within specific developmental stages. The developmental perspective discussed here should be distinguished from another use of the term found in the literature. This alternative definition refers to a sequence of development in the use of specific drugs. For example, the use of legal drugs typically precedes the use of illegal drugs.[75,76] Likewise, Kandel[3] stated that, "At least four *developmental* (italics added) stages in adolescent involvement in drugs can be identified:

1. Beer or wine;
2. Cigarettes and/or hard liquor;
3. Marijuana; and
4. Other illicit drugs." (p. 258)

One step toward a more qualitative approach to prevention education has been taken by Sameroff[77] and Sameroff and Chandler[78] who described a transactional model of substance abuse based on the development of the child within both a social and family context. Using the transactional framework, they outlined developmental factors from early childhood through adolescence that should be considered in identifying children and adolescents who are at risk for engaging in substance use and other risky behaviors.

Unfortunately, the transactional model lacks adequate definitions of appropriate age groupings ("stages")—a prerequisite for any truly qualitative model of abuse. Russac and Weaver[74] suggested that a good first approximation to a stage theory of substance use can be obtained by drawing on established theories of moral and cognitive development.[79–81] Theorists in these fields generally agree on the existence of three developmentally important periods: early childhood (4–6 yr of age), middle childhood (6–10 yr of age) and adolescence (10–18 yr of age). Although providing a useful starting point, this classification will certainly require "fine-tuning" as our knowledge about substance abuse among children and youth increases. For example, Russac and Weaver included *preadolescence* (10–12 yr of age) within the stage of adolescence. Yet we saw earlier that this period represents a time of exceptional vulnerability toward experimentation with a variety of drugs (*see* Table 1), and will almost certainly need to be targeted separately.

One ambitious and highly regarded developmentally-based model is found in work by Jessor[82] on problem-behavior proneness. A basic tenant of problem-behavior proneness is that a problem behavior is defined by its deviation from the norm. Moreover, norms are *age-graded.* Behavior becomes a problem when it appears at inappropriate times in the developmental sequence. To use a term borrowed from Neugarten and Hagestad,[83] problem behavior often results from *off-time events*—events that occur unusually early or unusually late, according to the social clock. Because drug-use behaviors (e.g., use of alcohol, cigarets, or marijuana) are often linked to progress from one developmental stage to the next, problem-behavior proneness equates to *transition-proneness* in the general developmental sense. That is, these behaviors mark a transition from childhood to adolescence or adolescence to young adulthood. Variables predictive of problem-behavior proneness include:

> . . . lower value on achievement and greater value on independence, greater social criticism, more tolerance of deviance, and less parental control and support, more friends' influence, and more friends' models and approval for drug use in the perceived environment system; more deviant behavior, less church attendance, lower school achievement in the behavior system. (pp. 132–133)[82]

One weakness of Jessor's model lies in the current lack of evidence showing clearly defined links between the variables identified by the model as indicative of problem-behavior proneness and specific group differences. In particular, these variables have not been adequately differentiated on the basis of gender.

Depth of Acceptance

One model currently being explored by the authors is a Depth of Acceptance (DOA) approach, which we have used to conceptualize a continuum of risk from vulnerability to immunity. The model rests on two assumptions: First, reasons for avoiding drug use range along a continuum from "shallow" acceptance, based entirely on external factors such as availability, to "deep" acceptance arising from a personal belief that drug use is wrong. Second, the deeper the level of acceptance, the more enduring and consistent an individual's immunity to drug use becomes. The DOA continuum, as presently conceived, consists of four "orientations." Moving from shallow to deep acceptance, they are:

An *external orientation* resides entirely in factors beyond the individual's control, such as availability of a drug, its cost, and the person's physical and financial ability to obtain it. This is the level of acceptance that drives most secondary prevention efforts, such as law enforcement and interdiction. The problem with an external orientation is that neither attitude nor behavior toward drug use has been altered. If drugs become available and affordable, the person will use them.

A second level of acceptance is *outcome orientation,* based on the perceived personal consequences of drug use. This type of message can be seen in the most recognizable prevention slogans, such as "This is your brain; this is your brain on drugs." Messages that warn of poor grades, harm to friends and family, ruined lives, incarceration, increased risk of accidents and violence, and both physical and psychological problems are outcome oriented. Within the context of the DOA model, outcome orientation, despite its widespread incorporation into prevention strategies, is hypothesized to be relatively ineffective in producing consistent long-term results. The weakness of outcome messages lies in their heavy reliance on threat of punishment, which learning theorists have long known to be less effective in changing behavior than reinforcing consequences. Skinner,[84] for example, believed that punishers merely suppress behavior rather than modify it. In his book, *Beyond Freedom and Dignity,* he wrote that punishment (or threat of punishment) is used on the " . . .assumption that a person who has been punished is less likely to behave in the same way again. Unfortunately, the matter is not that simple. Reward and punishment do not differ merely in the direction of the changes they induce. . . . Punished behavior is likely to reappear after the punitive contingencies are withdrawn" (p. 62).[84] Threat of punishment is akin to holding a club over a person's head; as long as the club is present, the behavior is suppressed; remove the club and the behavior returns.

A person's *social orientation* toward drug use is a function of the standards set and/or modeled by an adolescent's family, friends, peer groups, and role models. In this sense, the theoretical underpinnings of a social orientation are to be found in social learning theory as discussed earlier. We also expect social orientation to change systematically with development. Preschool children look primarily to their family for information about appropriate behavior. Youngsters in elementary school turn to people in authority, including parents, teachers, and other available role models. To a lesser extent, they also accept the standards of their same-sex playmates. Adolescents, of course, find their behavior standards primarily in the peer group.

The "deepest" level of acceptance is a *personal orientation,* a commitment that is maintained, despite external temptations and social pressures, because the individual personally believes that alcohol and other drug use is wrong. There are presently little clear data (or perhaps it would be more accurate to say there is a plethora of diverse and conflicting data) on how personal commitments are established. They may simply represent an over-identification with prevailing norms resulting from a single strong tie to a group or individual. Or they may be beliefs and behaviors instilled through exposure to a single, pervasive, continually reinforced set of standards across a variety of family, community, and social settings. Most significantly, personal commitments may require a pervasive restructuring and integration of an individual's entire attitude, value, and belief systems.

In a large factor analytic study of attitude items taken from the Duval Survey, support was found for three of the four orientations. Only a factor describing a personal orientation failed to emerge.[85] This may have resulted from the fact that only a single item describing a personal commitment to abstention from drug use is included in the survey. Scores for

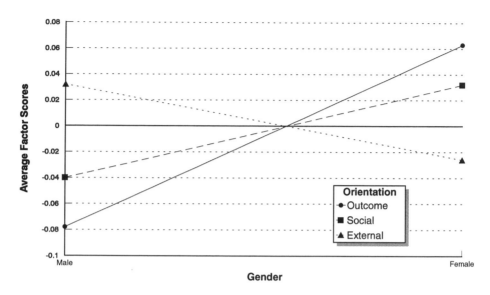

Fig. 2. "Depth of message" factor loadings.

each of the three factors were then subjected to one-way analyses of variance with grade, racial/ethnic background, and sex as classification variables. Although interesting patterns emerged for all three variables, gender differences are particularly revealing.

As seen in Fig. 2, males and females display contrasting patterns on all three orientations, with outcome and social orientations producing factor scores opposite those found for an external orientation. Female adolescents are most strongly influenced by outcome and socially oriented messages, a finding in line with previous research.[46] By contrast, male adolescents respond most strongly to messages based on external constraints. These differences in orientation toward drug use across gender may prove useful in fine-tuning drug prevention messages. We should emphasize, however, that no causal link between the factor patterns and actual resistance to drug use can be confirmed by these data. Still, we are sufficiently encouraged to have begun construction of an instrument designed specifically to measure DOA, one we hope will further refine the way we think about prevention and treatment messages conveyed to specific populations.

Conclusions

The unifying theme of this review can be summarized as follows: Those of us concerned with substance use among our youth can no longer be satisfied with a unitary approach to prevention and treatment. We can no longer hope to fight a war on drugs armed with only a single message, a single theory, or a single methodology. A prevention specialist should no longer feel comfortable walking into a large auditorium filled with young people intending to present a single antidrug message. Nor should a drug counselor be satisfied applying one treatment approach to all clients. Substance abuse is a complex phenomenon that requires complex solutions. In this chapter we have focused on female adolescents at risk for substance abuse—a population we believe have thus far been underserved since attention has focused on the more conspicuous problems of male substance abuse. However, the issue of selective identification and intervention is not limited to gender. Diversity, as Charles Darwin pointed out, is the rule rather than the exception.

References

[1]E. Adams, A. Blanken, L. Ferguson, and A. Kopstein (1990) *Overview of Selected Drug Trends*. National Institute on Drug Abuse, Rockville, MD.

[2]J. Shedler and J. Block (1990) Adolescent drug use and psychological health: a logical inquiry. *Am. Psychol.* **45,** 612–630.

[3]D. Kandel (1980) Drug and drinking behavior among youth. *Annu. Rev. Sociol.* **6,** 235–285.

[4]B. Bry (1978) Research design in drug abuse prevention: review and recommendations. *Int. J. Addict.* **13,** 1157–1168.

[5]S. Schinke and L. Gilchrist (1985) Preventing substance abuse with children and adolescents. *J. Consult. Clin. Psychol.* **53,** 596–602.

[6]M. Lavenhar (1979) Methodology in youth drug-abuse research, in *Youth Drug Abuse: Problems, Issues, and Treatment,* G. M. Beschner and A. S. Friedman, eds. Lexington Books, Toronto, pp. 113–128.

[7]M. Porter, T. Vieira, G. Kaplan, J. Heesch, and A. Colyar (1973) Drug use in Anchorage, Alaska. *JAMA* **223,** 657–664.

[8] B. Rouse, N. Kozel, and L. Richards (1985) *Self-Report Methods of Estimating Drug Use.* National Institute on Drug Abuse (NIDA research monograph #57), Rockville, MD.

[9]P. Whitehead and R. Smart (1972) Validity and reliability of self-reported drug abuse. *Can. J. Criminol. Corrections* **14,** 83–89.

[10]J. Rittenhouse, ed. (1977) *The epidemiology of Heroin and Other Narcotics.* National Institute on Drug Abuse (NIDA research monograph #16), Rockville, MD.

[11]L. Hunt (1977) Prevalence of active heroin use in the United States, in *The Epidemiology of Heroin and Other Narcotics.* J. D. Rittenhouse, ed. National Institute on Drug Abuse, Rockville, MD, pp. 61–86.

[12]P. Owen and L. Nyberg (1983) Assessing alcohol and drug problems among adolescents: current practices. *J. Drug Educ.* **13,** 249–254.

[13]T. McLellan and R. Dembo (1992) *Center for Substance Abuse Treatment's (CSAT) Screening and Assessment of Alcohol and Other Drug (AOD)-Abusing Adolescents: The Recommendations of a Consensus Panel.* Center For Substance Abuse Treatment (DHHS [ADM No. 270-91-0007]), Rockville, MD.

[14]R. Tarter (1990) Evaluation and treatment of adolescent substance abuse: a decision tree method. *Am. J. Drug Alcohol Abuse* **16,** 1–46.

[15] American Psychiatric Association (1987) *Diagnostic and Statistical Manual of Mental Disorders* (3rd ed., rev.). Author, Washington, DC.

[16]R. Knot and J. O'Neill (1990) Sobering thoughts. *Tex. Res. Soc. Alcohol. Newsletter* **2(6),** 1.

[17]L. Johnston, P. O'Malley, and J. Bachman (1992) *Smoking, Drinking, and Illicit Drug Use Among American Secondary School Students, College Students, and Young Adults, 1975–1991,* vol. 1. National Institute on Drug Abuse, Rockville, MD.

[18]US Department of Health and Human Services (1991) *National Household Survey on Drug Abuse.* Author, Rockville, MD.

[19]R. Russac and S. Weaver (1992) *The Fifth Duval Survey: A Community-Wide Survey of Substance Use Among Duval County Youth.* University of North Florida, Jacksonville, FL.

[20]W. Riley, J. Barenie, P. Mabe, and D. Myers (1990) Smokeless tobacco use in adolescent females: prevalence and psychosocial factors among racial/ethnic groups. *J. Behav. Med.* **13,** 207–220.

[21]M. Greenspan (1983) *A New Approach to Women and Therapy.* McGraw-Hill, New York.

[22]J. Mondanaro (1989) *Chemically Dependent Women: Assessment and Treatment.* Heath, Lexington, MA.

[23]E. Peluso and L. Peluso (1988) *Women and Drugs: Getting Hooked, Getting Clean.* CompCare, Minneapolis, MN.

[24]T. Barton and L. Johnson (1987) *The Weekly Reader Survey on Drugs and Drinking.* Field Publications, Middletown, CT.

[25]S. Wilsnack and L. Beckman, eds. (1985) *Alcohol Problems in Women.* Guilford, New York.

[26]M. Sandmaier (1980) *The Invisible Alcoholic: Women and Alcohol Abuse in America.* McGraw-Hill, New York.

[27]S. LeSourd (1987) *The Compulsive Woman.* Revell, Old Tappan, NJ.

[28]J. Schenker (1990) The risk of alcohol intake in men and women: all may not be equal. *N. Engl. J. Med.* **322,** 290–297.

[29]E. Gordis (1990) Alcohol and women: a commentary by NIAAA Enoch Gordis. *Alcohol Alert* **10,** 1–3.

[30]House Select Committee on Children, Youth, and Families (1990) *Getting Straight: Overcoming Treatment Barriers for Addicted Women and Their Children.* Hearing before the Select Committee, US Government Printing Office, Washington, DC.

[31]B. Reed (1987) Developing women-sensitive drug dependence treatment services: why so difficult? *J. Psychoactive Drugs* **19,** 151–164.

[32]J. Kagle (1986) Women who drink: changing images, changing realities. *J. Soc. Work Educ.* **23,** 21–28.

[33]J. Turnbull (1988) Primary and secondary alcoholic women. *Soc. Casework: J. Contemp. Soc. Work* **69,** 290–297.

[34]L. Robe (1986) *Co-Starring Famous Women Scholars.* Springer, New York.

[35]S. Wilsnack (1973) Sex role identity in female alcoholism. *J. Abnorm. Psychol.* **82,** 253–261.

[36]W. McCord and J. McCord (1959) *Origins of Crime.* Columbia University Press, New York.

[37]T. Hirschi (1969) *Causes of Delinquency.* University of California Press, Berkeley, CA.

[38]Hearing before the Committee on the Judiciary United States Senate (1992) *Cocaine Kindergartners: Preparing for the First Wave.* 102 Congress, 1st session, US Government Printing Office, Washington, DC.

[39]C. Mowbray, S. Lanir, and M. Hulce, eds. (1984) *Women and Mental Health: New Directions for Change.* Haworth, New York.

[40]M. Nichols (1985) Theoretical concerns in the clinical treatment of substance abusing women: a feminist analysis. *Alcohol Treatment Q.* **2(1),** 89–95.

[41]K. Fejes-Mendoza (1990) Drug exposed infants: outlook for educators, in *Mountain Plains Information Bulletin.* Drake University, Des Moines, IA.

[42]B. Mooney (1993) Special needs of dually diagnosed adolescent females. *Counselor* **11(3),** 21–24.

[43]B. Havassy, S. Hall, and D. Wasserman (1991) Social support and relapse: commonalities among alcoholics, opiate users, and cigarette smokers. *Addict. Behav.* **16,** 235–246.

[44]H. Weiner, M. Wallen, and G. Zankowski (1990) Culture and social class as intervening variables in relapse prevention with chemically dependent women. *J. Psychoactive Drugs* **22,** 239–248.

[45]E. Young (1990) The role of incest in relapse. *J. Psychoactive Drugs* **22,** 249–258.

[46]R. Jessor, S. Jessor, and J. Finney (1973) A social psychology of marijuana use: longitudinal studies of high school and college youth. *J. Personality Soc. Psychol.* **26,** 1–15.

[47]D. Kandel (1980) A second look at convergencies in longitudinal drug studies: an update, in *Epidemiology of Drug Abuse.* L. Robins, ed. WHO, Geneva, pp. 897–912.

[48]E. Erikson (1963) *Childhood and Society.* Norton, New York.

[49]L. Robins and E. Wish (1977) Childhood deviance as a developmental process: a study of 223 urban black men from birth to 18. *Soc. Forces* **56,** 448–471.

[50]A. DeLeon and N. Jainchill (1991) Residential therapeutic communities for female substance abusers. *Bull. NY Acad. Med.* **67,** 277–290.

[51]E. S. Linsansky-Gomberg (1989) Suicide risk among women with alcohol problems. *Am. J. Public Health* **79,** 1363–1365.

[52]R. Peveler and C. Fairburn (1990) Eating disorders in women who abuse alcohol. *Br. J. Addict.* **85,** 1633–1638.

[53]N. Finkelstein (1987) *Effects of Parental Alcoholism, Family Violence and Social Support on the Inter-Generational Transmission of Alcoholism in Adult Women.* Doctoral dissertation, Heller School, Brandeis University, Naltham, MA.

[54]E. Gomberg (1980) Risk factors related to alcohol problems among women: proneness and vulnerability, in *Alcohol and Women: Research Monograph No. One.* US Government Printing Office (HEW Publ. No. [ADM] 80-8-35), Washington, DC.

[55]N. Jainchill, G. DeLeon, and L. Pinkham (1986) Psychiatric diagnosis among substance abusers in therapeutic community treatment. *J. Psychoactive Drugs* **18,** 209–213.

[56]E. Corrigan (1980) *Alcoholic Women in Treatment.* Oxford University Press, New York.

[57]N. Finkelstein and E. Piedade (1993) The relational model and the treatment of addicted women. *Counselor* **11(3),** 8–12.

[58]D. Kandel (1973) Adolescent marijuana use: role of parents and peers. *Science* **181,** 1067–1070.

[59]D. Kandel, R. Kessler, and R. Margulies (1978) Antecedents of adolescent initiation into stages of drug use: a developmental analysis, in *Longitudinal Research on Drug Use.* D. Kandel, ed. Wiley, New York, pp. 73–99.

[60]T. Berndt (1979) Developmental changes in conformity to peers and parents. *Dev. Psychol.* **15,** 608–616.

[61]H. Swadi (1992) Relative risk factors in detecting adolescent drug use. *Drug Alcohol Dep.* **29,** 253,254.

[62]W. Lucas, S. Grupp, and R. Schmitt (1975) Predicting who will turn on: a four-year follow-up. *Int. J. Addict.* **10,** 305–326.

[63]R. Margulies, R. Kessler, and D. Kandel (1977) A longitudinal study of onset of drinking among high school students. *Q. J. Stud. Alcohol* **38,** 897–912.

[64]V. Bixenstine, M. DeCorte, and B. Bixenstine (1976) Conformity to peer-sponsored misconduct at four age levels. *Dev. Psychol.* **12,** 226–236.

[65]E. Devereux (1970) The role of the peer group experience in moral development, in *Minnesota Symposium on Child Psychology,* vol. 4. J. P. Hill, ed. University of Minnesota Press, Minneapolis, MN.

[66]M. Frezza, C. DiPadova, G. Pozzato, M. Terpin, E. Baraona, and C. Lieber (1990) High blood alcohol levels in women: the role of decreased gastric alcohol dehydrogenase and first pass metabolism. *N. Engl. J. Med.* **322,** 95–99.

[67]B. Streett (1993) Chemically dependent women and premenstrual syndrome. *Counselor* **11(3),** 18–20.

[68]S. Wilsnack, A. Klassen, and R. Wilsnack (1984) Drinking and reproductive dysfunction among women in a 1981 national survey. *Alcohol. Clin. Exp. Res.* **8,** 451–458.

[69]B. Skinner (1974) *About Behaviorism.* Knopf, New York.

[70]R. Akers (1977) *Deviant Behavior: Social Learning Approach* (2nd ed.). Wadsworth, Belmont, CA.

[71]R. Burgess and R. Akers (1966) A differential association-reinforcement theory of criminal behavior. *Soc. Probl.* **14,** 128–147.

[72]R. Akers, M. Krohn, L. Lanza-Kaduce, and M. Radosevich (1979) Social learning and deviant behavior: a specific test of a general theory. *Am. Soc. Rev.* **44,** 635–655.

[73]A. Bandura (1977) *Social Learning Theory.* Prentice-Hall, Englewood Cliffs, NJ.

[74]R. Russac and S. Weaver (1994) Fine-tuning the prevention message: a developmental perspective. *J. Alcohol/Drug Educ.* **39,** 46–55.

[75]D. Kandel (1975) Stages in adolescent involvement in drug use. *Science* **190,** 912–914.

[76]D. Kandel and R. Faust (1975) Sequences and stages in patterns of adolescent drug use. *Arch. Gen. Psychiatry* **32,** 923–932.

[77]A. J. Sameroff (1987) Transactional risk factors and prevention, in *Preventing Mental Disorders: A Research Perspective.* J. A. Steinberg and M. M. Silverman, eds. US Department of Health and Human Services (USDHHS Publication No. [ADM] 87-1492), Rockville, MD, pp. 74–89.

[78]A. J. Sameroff and M. J. Chandler (1975) Reproductive risks and the continuum of caretaking casualty, in *Review of Child Development Research.* F. D. Horowitz, M. Hetherington, S. Scarr-Salapatek, and G. Siegel, eds. University of Chicago, Chicago, pp. 87–244.

[79]L. Kohlberg (1976) Moral stages and moralization, in *Moral Development and Behavior: Theory, Research and Social Issues.* T. Lakona, ed. Holt, Rinehart and Winston, New York, pp. 31–53.

[80]J. Piaget (1932) *The Moral Judgment of the Child* (M. Gabain, trans.). Kegan, Paul, Trench, Trubner, London.

[81]J. Piaget (1967) *Six Psychological Studies.* Random House, New York.

[82]R. Jessor (1976) Predicting time of onset of marijuana use: a developmental study of high school youth. *J. Consult. Clin. Psychol.* **44,** 125–134.

[83]B. Neugarten and G. Hagestad (1976) Age in the life course, in *Handbook of Aging in the Social Sciences.* R. H. Binstock and E. Shanas, eds. Van Nostrand Reinhold, New York, pp. 35–55.

[84]B. Skinner (1971) *Beyond Freedom and Dignity.* Knopf, New York.

[85]R. Russac, S. Weaver, J. Harvard, and J. Hoagland (1994) *Reasons Adolescents Don't Use Drugs: Exploring a "Depth of Acceptance" Model.* Manuscript under revision.

Index